Kama

6 Boo

OVER 200+ Illustrated Sex
Beginners, Positions for Couples, Sex Games Guide, Tantric Sex, Foreplay & Dirty Talk.

Master Love & Seduction Secrets.

Lana Fox

COPYRIGHT

Table of Contents

First Book: HOW TO TALK DIRTY

INTRODUCTION

Since one of the most significant things in a relationship is correspondence, it possibly bodes well that when things get hot and overwhelming, you should keep on having an exchange. Indeed, I'm proposing dirty talk, and honestly, if you haven't checked out it during sex or foreplay, now is the right time. It's in reality not so terrifying.

While there are a lot of incredible articles out there about how to talk dirty to your accomplice, there aren't sufficient out there regarding why you ought to do it. The majority of these previously mentioned articles (not Bustle's obviously) are calculated such that you should talk to dirty to "your man," because that is "the thing that he enjoys," and needs, and the remainder of the heteronormative garbage that neglects to incorporate everybody. However, what those pieces appear to overlook is that when you carry dirty talk in with the general mish-mash, it isn't just about your accomplice and their needs; it's similarly about what you appreciate, as well, and a ton of us genuinely love to talk dirty. It feels great to allow everything to out.

Regardless of whether you decide to talk dirty in bed, using sexting, or like to enjoy classic telephone sex, talking dirty is undoubtedly something everybody should attempt. Here are eight hot reasons why.

1. It Helps You Learn What you're Comfortable With

The explanation there are such a significant number of articles about how to talk dirty is because it very well may be dubious from the outset. It can cause a few people to feel helpless against put themselves out there in such a vocal way. Afterward, there are the individuals who can't state certain words, similar to "pussy," or "cockerel," which, to be completely forthright, are the words you're often going for when you're talking dirty.

There's likewise the test of beating how you see words in reality and how your view them in the room. As sex advisor Vanessa Marin's segment for Bustle on talking dirty clarifies, it's OK to be turned by words like "prostitute," even though you may discover them hostile outside the room. You're assuming responsibility for the word and utilizing it on your standing, and that can be trying for certain ladies. Be that as it may, some of the time, a test encourages you characterize what you're OK with — on your terms.

2. It Keeps Your Partner In The Loop

Except if you're dating a mystic, you're accomplice can't guess what you might be thinking. When you vocalize what feels better, what needs some work, or that your clitoris is only somewhat higher, and you'd truly love it if your accomplice could concentrate all their vitality there, then you both advantages.

When you can both say what you like and how you like it, you're not very far away from saying how it affects you. From that point, the dirty talk will simply stream – it will take practice however.

3. It Gets Your Creative Juices (And Other Juices) Flowing

Along these lines, perhaps your rendition of talking dirty right presently is telling your accomplice that you're going to come. That is generally one part of dirty talk that individuals can handle, yet simply consider how hot it would be to simply let free and uncover all the things you keep in your mind during sex.

Before you know it, you've gone from hollering, "I'm coming! I'm coming!" to something about how you're going to appear at your accomplice's work, lock them in their office, and give them the sort of mid-day break that you've both needed continuously. At that time you've made a dream and a situation that you can hold returning to and can expand upon. Perhaps you'll even wind up receiving your adaptation of Fifty Shades of Gray in return – you never know!

4. It's Awesome Foreplay

As any specialist or sex advisor will let you know, foreplay is a critical piece of sex, particularly for ladies. It takes ladies far longer to get stirred than men, and that is the reason they don't climax as fast as men do. For us, foreplay is essential.

If you can begin with some dirty talk, then you'll be enticing each other in manners that are similarly as significant as physical foreplay. Quick ones are fun, yet if you have the opportunity to take as much time as is needed, then do it. Put aside an entire 20 minutes of simply talking dirty to one another before you even take off your garments and contact one another. You'll see the difference it makes.

5. You'll Surprise Yourself

It's always pleasant when you can even now astound yourself, right? Furthermore, the thing is, when you drive yourself to accomplish something that you've never done, you very well might understand it was made for you. Talking graphically about how you need to be contacted and how you're going to contact your accomplice may upset your sexual coexistence. However you'll ever discover except if you check out it.

6. You'll Surprise Your Partner

There are a lot of approaches to zest things up in your long haul relationship when things are feeling somewhat stale. If your sexual coexistence has become the stuff of evangelist directly before bed, then talking dirty to your accomplice is a simple method to change it up a piece.

Odds are the dirty things you've been thinking, yet haven't said so anyone can hear yet, will amaze them. You can murmur in your accomplice's ear, ensuring your lips just marginally brush their ear cartilage. From that point, contingent upon their reaction, you can proceed, or let them dominate and mention to you what they're thinking, as well.

7. It Leads To Better Sex

If you're talking honestly, transparently, and graphically about what you need to escape each sexual experience, in what manner can it not prompt better sex? With correspondence and so much dirty discussion, there are no insider facts — and neither you nor your accomplice is compelled to attempt to make sense of what that groan or outward appearance truly implies. Sex shouldn't be an enigma.

8. It's Fun (And Funny) As Hell

You may imagine that you must be genuine when you're talking dirty, yet you don't. A great deal of times, individuals overlook that in addition to the fact that sex is fun — it very well may be amusing, as well. If you can release up enough to make some great memories, snicker about it, and unwind, you'll be amazed by what kind of good time you can have.

I can't disclose to you the amount of my dirty talk has spun around pizza. I figure if there's no snickering in there sooner or later, then we've quite recently paid attention to ourselves as well. What's more, that is not hot.

WHY TOO MANY PEOPLE HAVE ROTTEN SEX LIVES

These ought to be blast times for sex.

The portion of Americans who state sex between unmarried grown-ups is "not off-base by any stretch of the imagination" is at an untouched high. New instances of HIV are at an untouched low. Most ladies can—finally—gain birth power for nothing, and a next day contraceptive without a solution.

If hookups are your thing, Grindr and Tinder offer the possibility of easygoing sex inside the hour. The expression If something exists, there is pornography of it used to be an astute web image; presently it's a cliché. BDSM plays at the nearby multiplex—however why trouble going? Sex is depicted, often graphically and here and there perfectly, on prime-time link. Sexting is, factually, ordinary.

Polyamory is a family unit word. Disgrace loaded terms like corruption have offered approach to chipper sounding ones like crimp. Butt-centric sex has gone from definite unthinkable to "fifth base"— Teen Vogue (indeed, Teen Vogue) even ran a manual for it. Except for maybe interbreeding and savagery—and nonconsensual sex all the more for the most part—our way of life has never been increasingly tolerant of sex in pretty much every stage.

However, notwithstanding this, American youngsters and youthful grown-ups are having less sex.

To the alleviation of numerous guardians, instructors, and pastorate individuals who care about the wellbeing and prosperity of youngsters, teenagers are propelling their sexual experiences later. From 1991 to 2017, the Centers for Disease Control and Prevention's Youth Risk Behavior Survey finds, the level of secondary school understudies who'd engaged in sexual relations dropped from 54 to 40 percent. In about an age, sex has gone from something most secondary school understudies have encountered to something most haven't. (What's more, no, they aren't having oral sex instead—that rate hasn't changed a lot.)

In the interim, the U.S. youngster pregnancy rate has plunged to 33% of its advanced high. When this decrease began, during the 1990s, it was broadly and adequately grasped. Be that as it may, presently a few eyewitnesses are starting to ponder whether an unambiguously beneficial thing may have establishes in less salubrious improvements. Signs are gathering that the deferral in high schooler sex may have been the principal sign of a more extensive withdrawal from physical closeness that broadens well into adulthood.

In recent years, Jean M. Twenge, a brain science teacher at San Diego State University, has distributed research investigating how and why Americans' sexual experiences might be ebbing. In a progression of diary articles and her most recent book, iGen, she takes note of that the present youthful grown-ups are on target to have less sex accomplices than individuals from the two going before ages. Individuals now in their mid 20s are more than multiple times as prone to be abstinent as Gen Xers were at that age; 15 percent report having had no sex since they arrived at adulthood.

Gen Xers and Baby Boomers may likewise be having less sex today than past ages did at a similar age. From the late 1990s to 2014, Twenge discovered, drawing on information from the General Social Survey, the average grown-up went from engaging in sexual relations 62 times each year to multiple times. A given individual probably won't notice this reduction, yet broadly, it means a great deal of missing sex. Twenge as of late investigated the most recent General Social Survey information, from 2016, and revealed to me that in the two years following her examination, sexual recurrence fell much further.

Some social researchers disagree with parts of Twenge's investigation; others state that her information source, albeit exceptionally respected, isn't undeniably fit to sex inquire about. But none of the numerous specialists I met for this piece genuinely tested that the average youthful grown-up around 2018 is having less sex than their partners of decades past. Nor did anybody question that this the truth is out of venture with open recognition—a large portion of us despite everything feel that others are having significantly more sex than they are.

When I called the anthropologist Helen Fisher, who studies love and sex and co-coordinates Match.com's yearly Singles in America overview of more than 5,000 unpartnered Americans, I could nearly feel her gesturing via telephone. "The information is that individuals are having less sex," she stated, with a trace of naughtiness. "I'm a Baby Boomer, and clearly in my day we were having significantly more sex than they are today!" She proceeded to clarify that the study has been testing the personal subtleties of individuals' lives for a long time now. "Consistently the entire Match organization is fairly stumbled at how little sex Americans are having—including the Millennials."

Fisher, in the same way as other different specialists, credits the sex decay to a decrease in couplehood among youngsters. For 25 years, less individuals have been wedding, and the individuals who do have been wedding later. From the start, numerous spectators calculated that the decrease in marriage was clarified by an expansion in unmarried living together—yet the portion of individuals living respectively hasn't sufficiently risen to balance the decrease in marriage: About 60 percent of grown-ups under age 35 presently live without a life partner or an accomplice. One out of three grown-ups right now live with their folks, making that the most widely recognized living course of action for the partner. Individuals who live with a sentimental accomplice will in general engage in sexual relations more than the individuals who don't—and living with your folks is awful for your sexual coexistence. However, this doesn't clarify why youngsters are collaborating up less in any case.

Throughout numerous discussions with sex scientists, analysts, financial analysts, sociologists, advisors, sex instructors, and youthful grown-ups, I heard numerous different hypotheses about what I have come to consider as the sex downturn. I was told it may be a result of the hookup culture, of smashing financial weights, of flooding tension rates, of mental delicacy, of across the board stimulant use, of spilling TV, of natural estrogens spilled by plastics, of dropping testosterone levels, of computerized pornography, of the vibrator's brilliant age, of dating applications, of choice loss of motion, of helicopter guardians, of careerism, of cell phones, of the sequence of media reports, of data over-burden for the most part, of lack of sleep, of stoutness. Name a cutting edge curse, and somebody, some place, is prepared to reprimand it for disturbing the advanced charisma.

A few specialists I talked with offered increasingly cheerful clarifications for the decrease in sex. For instance, paces of youth sexual maltreatment have diminished in late decades, and misuse can prompt both gifted and unbridled sexual conduct. Also, a few people today may feel less compelled into sex they would prefer not to have, because of changing sex mores and developing attention to assorted sexual directions, including asexuality. Possibly more individuals are organizing school or work over adoration and sex, at any rate for a period, or perhaps they're being extra intentional in picking a life accomplice—and if along these lines, bravo.

Many—or all—of these things might be valid. In a celebrated 2007 examination, individuals provided analysts with 237 particular explanations behind engaging in sexual relations, running from magical ("I needed to feel nearer to God") to faltering ("I needed to change the subject of discussion"). The quantity of reasons not to engage in sexual relations must be at any rate as high. In any case, a bunch of suspects came up over and over in my meetings and the exploration I evaluated—and every ha significant ramifications for our joy.

1. Sex for One

The retreat from sex isn't a solely American marvel. Most nations don't follow their residents' sexual experiences intently, however those that attempt (every one of them affluent) are announcing their sex postponements and decays. One of the most regarded sex considers on the planet, Britain's National Survey of Sexual Attitudes and Lifestyles, detailed in 2001 that individuals ages 16 to 44 were having intercourse over six times each month by and large. By 2012, the rate had dropped to less than multiple times. Over generally a similar period, Australians seeing someone went from engaging in sexual relations about 1.8 times each week to 1.4 occasions. Finland's "Finsex" study discovered decreases in intercourse recurrence, alongside rising paces of masturbation.

In the Netherlands, the middle age at which individuals initially engage in sexual relations rose from 17.1 in 2012 to 18.6 in 2017, and different kinds of physical contact additionally got pushed back, kissing. This news was welcomed not with all inclusive alleviation, as in the United States, however with some worry. The Dutch value having a portion of the world's most elevated paces of immature and youthful grown-up prosperity. If individuals skirt a urgent period of advancement, one teacher cautioned—a phase that incorporates being a tease and kissing as well as managing shock and disillusionment—may they be not ready for the difficulties of grown-up life?

Then, Sweden, which hadn't done a national sex study in 20 years, as of late propelled one, frightened by surveying proposing that Swedes, as well, were having less sex. The nation, which has one of the most noteworthy birth rates in Europe, is unwilling to hazard its fertility. "If the social conditions for a decent sexual coexistence—for instance through pressure or other unfortunate elements—have weakened," the Swedish wellbeing pastor at the time wrote in a commentary clarifying the method of reasoning for the examination, it is "a political issue."

This carries us to ripeness tested Japan, which is amidst a segment emergency and has become something of a contextual analysis in the threats of sexlessness. In 2005, 33% of Japanese single individuals ages 18 to 34 were virgins; by 2015, 43 percent of individuals right now were, and the offer who said they didn't mean to get hitched had risen as well. (Not excessively marriage was any assurance of sexual recurrence: A related review found that 47 percent of married individuals hadn't had intercourse in at any rate a month.)

For almost 10 years, stories in the Western press have attached Japan's sexual funk to a rising age of soushoku danshi—actually, "grass-eating young men." These "herbivore men," as they are known in English, are said to be hesitant about seeking after either ladies or ordinary achievement. The new scientific classification of Japanese sexlessness additionally incorporates terms for gatherings, for example, hikikomori ("shut-ins"), parasaito shinguru ("parasite singles," individuals who live with their folks past their 20s), and otaku ("over the top fans," particularly of anime and manga)— every one of whom are said to add to sekkusu shinai shokogun ("abstinence disorder").

From the get-go, most Western records of this had a substantial subtext of "Isn't Japan wacky?" This tone has gradually offered path to an acknowledgment that the nation's experience may be less an oddity than a useful example. Inauspicious business possibilities assumed an underlying job in driving numerous men to single interests—however the way of life has since moved to oblige and even support those interests. Roland Kelts, a Japanese

American essayist and long-lasting Tokyo inhabitant, has depicted "an age that found the defective or simply sudden requests of true associations with ladies less tempting than the draw of the virtual drive."

How about we think about this bait for a minute. Japan is among the world's top makers and shoppers of pornography, and the originator of entirely different pornography classes, for example, bukkake (don't inquire). It is additionally a worldwide innovator in the structure of top of the line sex dolls. What might be additionally telling, however, is the degree to which Japan is concocting methods of genital incitement that never again trouble to inspire old-fashioned sex, by which I mean sex including more than one individual. An ongoing article in The Economist, titled "Japan's Sex Industry Is Becoming Less Sexual," portrayed onakura shops, where men pay to stroke off. At the same time, female representatives watch, and clarified that because numerous more youthful individuals consider the to be thought of intercourse as mendokusai—tedious—"administrations that make masturbation progressively charming are blasting."

In their 2015 book, Modern Romance, the humanist Eric Klinenberg and the entertainer Aziz Ansari (who not long ago got scandalous for a hookup gone astray) depict Ansari's visit to Japan looking for bits of knowledge into the fate of sex. He presumed that a lot of what he'd read about herbivore men came up short. Herbivores, he found, were "keen on sexual joy"— only not "through conventional courses." Among Japan's increasingly well-known ongoing developments, he notes, is "a solitary use silicone egg that men load up with ointment and jerk off inside." One night in Tokyo, Ansari gets one a comfort store, goes to his lodging, and—sorry for the visual—gives it a go. He thinks that its cold and unbalanced, yet comprehends its motivation. "It was a way," he expresses, "to abstain from putting yourself out there and having a genuine encounter with someone else."

From 1992 to 2014, the portion of American men who revealed jerking off in a given week multiplied, to 54 percent, and the portion of ladies dramatically multiplied, to 26 percent. Simple access to pornography is a piece of the story, obviously; in 2014, 43 percent of men said they'd watched pornography in the previous week. The vibrator figures in, as well—a significant report 10 years prior found that simply over portion of grown-up ladies had utilized one, and by all signs it has just developed in notoriety. (Makes, models, and highlights have certainly increased. If you don't have the foggiest idea about your Fun Factory Bi Stronic Fusion pulsator from your Power Toyfriend, you can discover them on Amazon, which has these and somewhere in the range of 10,000 different choices.)

This shift is especially striking when you consider that Western human progress has had a significant hang-up about masturbation returning at any rate similarly as Onan. As Robert T. Michael and his co-creators relate in Sex in America, J. H. Kellogg, the oat creator, asked American guardians of the late nineteenth century to take outrageous measures to shield their kids from reveling, including circumcision without sedative and utilization of carbolic corrosive to the clitoris. Much obliged to a limited extent to his message, masturbation stayed unthinkable well into the twentieth century. By the 1990s, when Michael's book turned out, references to masturbation were still welcomed with "anxious titters or with stun and appall," notwithstanding the way that the conduct was typical.

Today, masturbation is significantly progressively normal, and fears about its belongings—presently matched with worries about computerized pornography's universality—are being raised again by an abnormal collection of individuals, including the therapist Philip Zimbardo, the chief of the well-known Stanford Prison Experiment, who is getting a charge out of a far-fetched second go about as an antiporn lobbyist. In his book Man, Interrupted, Zimbardo cautions that "procrasturbation"— his grievous portmanteau for delaying using masturbation—might be driving youngsters to bomb scholastically, socially, and explicitly. Gary Wilson, an Oregon man who runs a site called Your Brain on Porn, makes a comparative case. In a mainstream tedx talk, which highlights creature sexual intercourse just as many (human) cerebrum examines, Wilson contends that stroking off to web pornography is addictive, causes fundamental changes in the mind, and is delivering a plague of erectile brokenness.

These messages are resounded and amplified by a Salt Lake City–based charitable considered Fight the New Drug—the "medicate" being pornography—which has conveyed several introductions to schools and different associations around the nation, including, this spring, the Kansas City Royals. The site NoFap, a branch of a well known Reddit message board established by a presently resigned Google contractual worker, gives network individuals ("fapstronauts") a program to stop "fapping"— stroking off. Further outside the standard, the extreme right Proud Boys bunch has a "no wanks" strategy, which precludes jerking off more than once per month. The gathering's organizer, Gavin McInnes, who additionally helped to establish Vice Media, has said that erotic entertainment and masturbation are making Millennials "not have any desire to seek after connections."

Reality shows up increasingly convoluted. There is insufficient proof of a scourge of erectile brokenness among youngsters. Furthermore, no analyst I talked with had seen convincing proof that pornography is addictive. As the creators of an ongoing survey of pornography explore note in The Archives of Sexual Behavior, "The thought of tricky sex entertainment use stays disagreeable in both scholarly and famous writing." At the same time "the emotional well-being network everywhere is isolated with regards to the addictive versus non-addictive nature of Internet sex entertainment."

This isn't to state there's no relationship between's pornography use and want for genuine sex. Ian Kerner, a notable New York sex specialist and the writer of a few well known books about sex, revealed to me that while he doesn't see pornography use as undesirable (he prescribes specific kinds of pornography to certain patients), he works with a great deal of men who, propelled by pornography, "are as yet jerking off like they're 17," to the burden of their sexual coexistence. "It's offering some relief from their craving," he said. Kerner accepts this is the reason increasingly more of the ladies going to his office as of late report that they need sex more than their accomplices do.

In detailing this story, I talked and related with many 20-and mid-30-somethings with expectations of better understanding the sex downturn. I can't realize that they were agent, however I sought out individuals with a scope of encounters. I talked with some who had never had a sentimental or sexual relationship, and other people who were fiercely enamored or had occupied sexual experiences or both. Sex might be declining, yet a great many people are as yet having it—in any event, during a financial downturn, a great many people are utilized.

The downturn illustration is blemished. A great many people need occupations; that is not the situation with connections and sex. I talked with a lot of individuals who were single and chaste by decision. All things being equal, I was surprised by what number of twenty-year-olds were profoundly discontent with the sex-and-dating scene; again and again, individuals asked me whether things had consistently been this hard. Despite the decent variety of their accounts, specific topics rose.

One repeating topic, typically enough, was pornography. Less expected, maybe, was the degree to which numerous individuals saw their pornography life and their sexual coexistence as altogether separate things. The divider between the two was not total; for a specific something, numerous straight ladies disclosed to me that finding out about sex from pornography appeared to have given a few men overwhelming sexual propensities. (We'll find a workable pace.) But overall, the two things—cooperated sex and lone pornography seeing—existed on discrete planes. "My pornography taste and accomplice taste are very different," one man in his mid-30s let me know, clarifying that he watches pornography about once per week and doesn't think it has a lot of impact on his sexual coexistence. "I watch it realizing it is fiction," a 22-year-elderly person stated, including that she didn't "disguise" it.

I thought of these remarks when Pornhub, the top sex entertainment site, discharged its rundown of 2017's most mainstream look. In the lead position, for the third year running, was lesbian (a classification cherished by people the same). The new next in line, be that as it may, was hentai—anime, manga, and other animated pornography. Pornography has never been similar to genuine sex however hentai isn't even of this world; falsity is the wellspring of its intrigue. In a New York–magazine main story on pornography inclinations, Maureen O'Connor depicted the ways hentai transmogrifies body parts ("eyes greater than feet, bosoms the size of heads, penises thicker than abdomens") and eroticizes the powerful ("hot human shapes" consolidate with "sweets hued hide and creature horns, ears, and tails"). The main quest classification for pornography includes sex that a large portion of the populace doesn't have the hardware to take part in, and the next in line isn't licentious to such an extent as illusory.

Huge numbers of the more youthful individuals I talked with consider pornography to be only one progressively computerized action—a method for calming pressure, a preoccupation. It is identified with their sexual coexistence (or scarcity in that department) similarly web-based social networking and marathon watching TV are. As one 24-year-elderly person messaged me:

The web has made it so natural to gratify fundamental social and sexual needs that there's far less motivating force to go out into the "meatworld" and pursue those things. It is not necessarily the case that the web can give you more fulfillment than sex or connections, because it doesn't ... [But it can] supply you with merely enough fulfillment to appease those objectives ... I believe it's beneficial to ask yourself: "If I didn't have any of this, would I be going out additional? Would I engage in sexual relations more?" For many individuals my age, I think the appropriate response is most likely yes.

Indeed, even individuals seeing someone disclosed to me that their advanced life appeared to be competing with their sexual coexistence. "We'd presumably have much more sex," one lady noted, "if we didn't return home and turn on the TV and begin looking through our telephones." This appears to make no sense; our strive after sex should be base. Who might pick messing around online over genuine messing around?

Young people, for one. A charming examination distributed a year ago in the Journal of Population Economics inspected the presentation of broadband web access at the province by-district level, and found that its appearance disclosed 7 to 13 percent of the youngster birth-rate decrease from 1999 to 2007.

Possibly teenagers are not the hormone-crazed crazy people we some of the time describe them. Possibly the human sex drive is more delicate than we suspected, and all the more effectively slowed down.

2. Hookup Culture and Helicopter Parents

I began secondary school in 1992, around the time the youngster pregnancy and birth rates hit their most elevated levels in decades, and the middle age at which adolescents started having intercourse was moving toward its cutting edge low of 16.9. Ladies conceived in 1978, the year I was conceived, have a questionable respect: We were more youthful when we began engaging in sexual relations than any gathering since.

Be that as it may, as the '90s proceeded, the high schooler pregnancy rate started to decrease. This advancement was invited—regardless of whether specialists couldn't concur on why it was going on. Anti-conception medication advocates usually highlighted anti-conception medication. What's more, indeed, young people were showing signs of improvement about utilizing contraceptives, yet not adequately better to without any help clarify the change. Christian expert forbearance gatherings and sponsor of restraint just training, which got a significant subsidizing support from the 1996 government assistance change act, additionally attempted to assume praise. However the adolescent pregnancy rate was falling even in places that hadn't received restraint just educational plans, and research has since indicated that virginity vows and forbearance just training don't generate forbearance.

The pattern proceeded: Each rush of young people engaged in sexual relations somewhat later, and the pregnancy rate continued crawling down. You wouldn't have known both of these things, however, from all the hyperventilating about hookup culture that began in the late '90s. The New York Times, for instance, declared in 1997 that on school grounds, easygoing sex "is by all accounts close to an unequaled high." It didn't offer a lot of information to help this, however it introduced the paper's perusers to the term connecting, which it characterized as "anything from 20 minutes of strenuous kissing to going through the night together completely dressed to sex."

Basically from that point onward, individuals have been overestimating how much easygoing sex secondary school and understudies are having (even, reviews appear, understudies themselves). In the previous quite a while, be that as it may, various examinations and books on hookup culture have started to address the record. One of the most mindful of these is American Hookup: The New Culture of Sex on Campus, by Lisa Wade, a human science teacher at Occidental College. The book draws on nitty gritty diaries kept by understudies at two aesthetic sciences schools from 2010 to 2015, just as on Wade's discussions with understudies at 24 different universities and colleges.

Swim sorts the understudies she followed into three gatherings. Around 33% were what she calls "teetotalers"— they quit hookup culture altogether. Somewhat more than a third were "dilettantes"— they snared some of the time, yet irresolutely. Not precisely a quarter were "aficionados," who took pleasure in connecting. The rest of in long haul connections.

This picture is good with a recent report finding that Millennial undergrads weren't having more sex or sexual accomplices than their Gen X antecedents. It additionally follows information from the Online College Social Life Survey, an overview of in excess of 20,000 undergrads that was directed from 2005 to 2011, which found the middle number of hookups over a four-year school vocation to be five—33% of which included just kissing and contacting. Most of understudies reviewed said they wished they had more chances to locate a long haul sweetheart or sweetheart.

When I talked with Wade as of late, she disclosed to me that she found the sex decay among adolescents and twenty-year-olds obvious—youngsters, she stated, have consistently been well on the way to engage in sexual relations with regards to a relationship. "Return to the point in history where pre-marriage sex turned out to be to a greater degree a thing, and the conditions that prompted it," she stated, alluding to how post–World War II uneasiness about a man lack drove high schooler young ladies in the late 1940s and '50s to seek after more genuine sentimental connections than had been standard before the war. "Young ladies, by then, enhance 'going steady,' " Wade stated, including that guardians were not so much cheerful about the shift away from prewar romance, which had supported easygoing, nonexclusive dating. "If you [go out with somebody for] one night you may find a good pace smidgen of necking and petting, yet what happens when you go through months with them? It turns out 1957 has the most elevated pace of high schooler births in American history."

"We attach because we have no social abilities. We have no social abilities because we connect."

In later decades, on the other hand, youngster sentimental connections seem to have become less normal. In 1995, the enormous longitudinal examination known as "Include Health" found that 66 percent of 17-year-elderly people men and 74 percent of 17-year-elderly people ladies had encountered "a unique sentimental relationship" in the previous year and a half. In 2014, when the Pew Research Center asked 17-year-olds whether they had "ever dated, snared with or in any case had a sentimental relationship with someone else"—apparently a more extensive class than the previous one—just 46 percent said yes.

So what foiled adolescent sentiment? Pre-adulthood has changed such a considerable amount in the previous 25 years that it's difficult to tell where to begin. As Jean Twenge wrote in The Atlantic a year ago, the level of youngsters who report going on dates has diminished close by the rate who report different exercises related with entering adulthood, such as drinking liquor, working for pay, going out without one's folks, and getting a driver's permit.

These shifts concur with another significant change: guardians' expanded tension about their kids' instructive and financial possibilities. Among the well-to-do and instructed, mainly, this nervousness has prompted enormous changes in what's anticipated from adolescents. "It's difficult to work in sex when the baseball crew rehearses at 6:30, school begins at 8:15, show club meets at 4:15, the soup kitchen begins serving at 6, and, gracious no doubt, your screenplay needs fulfillment," said a man who was a few years out of school, recalling his secondary school years. He included: "There's huge weight" from guardians and other position figures "to concentrate on oneself, to the detriment of connections"— pressure, many twenty-year-olds let me know, that broadens directly on through school.

Malcolm Harris sends out a comparative vibe in his book, Kids These Days: Human Capital and the Making of Millennials. Tending to the desexing of the American youngster, he composes:

A decrease in solo available time presumably contributes a ton. At an essential level, sex at its best is unstructured play with companions, a class of experience that ... time journals ... let us know has been diminishing for American young people. It takes inert hands to move beyond a respectable starting point, and the present children have a ton to do.

Marriage 101, one of the most well-known college courses at Northwestern University, was propelled in 2001 by William M. Pinsof, an establishing father of couples treatment, and Arthur Nielsen, a psychiatry educator. Consider the possibility that you could instruct about affection, sex, and marriage before individuals picked an accomplice, Pinsof and Nielsen pondered—before they grew negative behavior patterns. The class was intended to be a kind of preemptive negative mark against miserable relationships. Under Alexandra Solomon, the brain science educator who assumed control over the course six years prior, it has become, optionally, a negative mark against what she sees as the sentimental and sexual hindering of an age. She doles out understudies to ask another person out on the town, for instance, something many have never done.

This hasn't hurt the class' allure; during enlistment, it fills in practically no time. (It could have helped that a course with covering claim, Human Sexuality, was ceased a few years back after its teacher managed an exhibit of something many refer to as a fucksaw.) Each week during available time, understudies hold up in line to talk with Solomon. He is likewise a rehearsing advisor at the college's Family Institute, about the class as well as about their affection troubles and all that they don't think about solid and pleasurable sex—which, as a rule, is a great deal.

Through the span of various discussions, Solomon has reached different decisions about hookup culture, or what may all the more precisely be portrayed as absence of-relationship culture. For a specific something, she trusts it is both a reason and an impact of social hindering. Or on the other hand, as one of her understudies put it to her: "We attach because we have no social aptitudes. We have no social aptitudes because we attach." For another, to the extent that her understudies wind up picking between easygoing sex and no sex, they are doing so because an undeniable third alternative—relationship sex—strikes huge numbers of them as unattainable as well as conceivably untrustworthy. Most Marriage 101 understudies have had at any rate one sentimental relationship through the span of their school vocation; the class usually pulls in relationship-situated understudies, she brings up. Regardless, she accepts that numerous understudies have retained that adoration is auxiliary to academic and expert achievement—or, at any rate, is best deferred until those different things have been made sure about. "Again and again," she has expressed, "my students reveal to me they make a decent attempt not to begin to look all starry eyed at during school, envisioning that would destroy their arrangements."

One Friday evening in March, I participated in a conversation Solomon was facilitating for a gathering of overwhelmingly female alumni understudies in the Family Institute's directing projects, on the difficulties of adoration and sex around 2018. Over rosé and brownies, understudies shared considerations on subjects extending from Aziz Ansari's infamous date (which had as of late been itemized on the site Babe) to the ambiguities of current relationship wording. "Individuals will resemble, 'We're dating, we're select, yet we're not beau and sweetheart.' What does that mean?" one young lady asked, exasperated. A cohort gestured unequivocally. "I don't get that's meaning? We're in a monogamous relationship, yet ... " She trailed off. Solomon hopped in with a kind of relationship litmus test: "If I get this season's cold virus, are you bringing me soup?" Around the gathering table, heads shook; very few individuals were getting (or giving) soup.

The discussion continued to why soup-bringing connections weren't increasingly normal. "You should have such a great amount before you can get into a relationship," one lady advertised. Another said that when she was in secondary school, her folks, who are the two experts with cutting edge degrees, had debilitated connections because they may decrease her core interest. Indeed, even today, in graduate school, she was finding the demeanor challenging to shake. "Presently I have to complete school, I have to get a work on moving, I have to do this and this, and afterward I'll consider love. In any case, by 30, you're similar to, What is love? What's it like to be infatuated?"

He was unable to get away from the feeling that hitting on somebody in person had, in a brief timeframe, gone from typical conduct to verge dreadful.

Toward the beginning of May, I came back to Northwestern to participate in a Marriage 101 conversation segment. I had picked that specific week because the assigned subject, "Sex in Intimate Relationships," appeared to be necessary. As it occurred, however, there wasn't a lot of talk of sex; the meeting was for the most part devoured by an upbeat discussion about the understudies' encounters with something many refer to as the "coach couple" task, which had included talking a couple in the network and chronicling their relationship.

"To see a relationship where two individuals are completely content and submitted," one lady stated, with genuine conviction, "it's sort of a moment of realization for me." Another understudy talked disbelievingly of her couple's pre-cell phone romance. "I couldn't identify with it," she said. "They met, they got each other's email addresses, they messaged each other, they went on a first date, they realized that they would have been as one. They never had a 'characterize the relationship' minute, because both were in agreement. I was much the same as, Damn, is that what it should resemble?" About 66% of the route through the distributed conversation time, one of the instructing collaborators at long last intruded. "Should we progress?" she asked, probably. "I needed to change to talk about sex. Which is the subject of this current week."

3. The Tinder Mirage

Simon, a 32-year-old graduate understudy who depicts himself as short and thinning up top ("If I weren't amusing," he says, "I'd be damned"), didn't need for sex in school. (The names of individuals who talked with me about their own lives have been transformed.) "I'm friendly and like to talk, yet I am on the most fundamental level a significant geek," he disclosed to me when we talked as of late. "I was glad to the point that school had geeky ladies. That was an enjoyment." Shortly before graduation, he began a relationship that went on for a long time. When he and his better half separated, in 2014, he was inclined that he'd ventured out of a time machine.

Before the relationship, Tinder didn't exist; nor did iPhones. Simon wasn't especially anxious to get into another genuine relationship immediately, however he needed to engage in sexual relations. "My first nature was go to bars," he said. Yet, each time he went to one, he struck out. He was unable to get away from the feeling that hitting on somebody in person had, in a brief timeframe, gone from ordinary conduct to verge dreadful. His companions set up a Tinder represent him; later, he pursued Bumble, Match, OkCupid, and Coffee Meets Bagel.

Except if you are incredibly attractive, the thing internet dating might be best at is sucking up a lot of time.

He would be wise to karma with Tinder than the different applications, yet it was not useful. He figures he swiped right—showing that he was intrigued—up to multiple times for each lady who additionally swiped directly on him, along these lines setting off a match. Be that as it may, coordinating was just the start; then the time had come to begin informing. "I was up to more than 10 messages sent for a solitary message got," he said. As it were: Nine out of 10 ladies who coordinated with Simon in the wake of swiping directly on him didn't proceed to trade messages with him. This implies for each 300 ladies he swiped right on, he discussed with only one.

At any rate among individuals who don't utilize dating applications, the observation exists that they encourage easygoing sex with exceptional effectiveness. In all actuality, except if you are especially gorgeous, the thing internet dating might be best at is sucking up a lot of time. Starting at 2014, when Tinder last discharged such information, the average client signed in 11 times each day. Men went through 7.2 minutes per meeting and ladies went through 8.5 minutes, for an aggregate of about 90 minutes every day. However they didn't receive much consequently. Today, the organization says it logs 1.6 billion swipes per day, and only 26 million matches. Also, if Simon's experience is any sign, the dominant part of matches don't prompt to such an extent as a two-way message trade, considerably less a date, significantly less sex.

When I talked with Simon, he was seven months into a relationship with another sweetheart, whom he'd met through another web based dating administration. He enjoyed her, and was glad to be on rest from Tinder. "It resembles crying into the void for most folks," he clarified, "and like looking for a jewel in an ocean of dick pics for most young ladies."

So for what reason do individuals keep on utilizing dating applications? Why not blacklist them all? Simon said meeting somebody disconnected appeared less and less of an alternative. His folks had met in a chorale a couple of years after school, however he was unable to see himself pulling off something comparative. "I play volleyball," he included. "I had someone on the volleyball crew two years back who I thought was adorable, and we'd been playing together for some time." Simon needed to ask her out, at the end of the day reasoned this would be "unimaginably cumbersome," even "animalistic."

From the outset, I pondered whether Simon was as a rule excessively respectable, or somewhat suspicious. However, the more individuals I talked with, the more I came to accept that he was essentially depicting a developing social reality. "Nobody approaches anybody in open any longer," said an instructor in Northern Virginia. "The dating scene has changed. Individuals are more reluctant to ask you out, all things considered, presently, or even talk in the first place," said a 28-year-elderly person in Los Angeles who chipped in that she had been single for a long time.

As sentiment and its beginnings are isolated from the schedules of everyday life, there is less and less space for lift tease.

This shift is by all accounts quickening amid the national retribution with rape and provocation, and an associative shifting of limits. As per a November 2017 Economist/YouGov survey, 17 percent of Americans ages 18 to 29 presently accept that a man welcoming a lady out for a beverage "consistently" or "for the most part" establishes inappropriate behavior. (Among more seasoned gatherings, a lot littler rates accept this.)

Laurie Mintz, who encourages a mainstream college course on the brain research of sexuality at the University of Florida, disclosed to me that the #MeToo development has made her understudies substantially more mindful of issues encompassing assent. She has gotten notification from numerous youngsters who are gainfully reconsidering their past activities and working industriously to gain from the encounters of companions and accomplices. Be that as it may, others have portrayed less sound responses, such as maintaining a strategic distance from sentimental suggestions for dread that they may be unwelcome. In my discussions, people the same talked about another uncertainty and aversion. One lady who portrayed herself as an energetic women's activist said she felt sympathy for the weight that hetero dating puts on men. "I think I owe it to them, right now minute especially, to attempt to treat them like they're individuals facing a challenge talking to a more abnormal," she thought of me. "There are a great deal of forlorn, befuddled individuals out there, who have no clue what to do or how to date."

I referenced to a few of the individuals I met for this piece I'd met my significant other in a lift, in 2001. (We dealt with different floors of a similar establishment, and throughout the months that followed started up a lot more discussions—in the lift, in the lounge, on the stroll to the tram.) I was captivated by the degree to which this provoked other ladies to moan and state that they'd simply love to meet somebody that way. But a significant number of them recommended that if an arbitrary person began talking to them in a lift, they would be weirded out. "Creeper! Escape from me," one lady envisioned reasoning. "Whenever we're peacefully, we take a gander at our telephones," clarified her companion, gesturing. Another lady fantasized to me about what it resembles to have a man hit on her in a book shop. (She'd hold a duplicate of her preferred book. "What's that book?" he'd state.) But then she appeared to wake up from her dream, and changed the subject to Sex and the City reruns and how miserably dated they appear. "Miranda meets Steve at a bar," she stated, in a tone recommending that the situation should be out of a Jane Austen epic, for all the pertinence it had to her life.

How could different dating applications be so wasteful at their apparent reason—attaching individuals—and still be so mainstream? For a certain something, heaps of individuals seem, by all accounts, to be utilizing them as a preoccupation, with constrained desires for meeting up face to face. As Iris, who's 33, let me know sharply, "They've gamified communication. Most of men on Tinder simply swipe directly on everyone. They state indeed, truly, yes to each lady."

Stories from other application clients substantiate the possibility of applications as preoccupations instead of relational arrangers. "Getting right-swiped is a decent inner self lift regardless of whether I have no aim of meeting somebody," one man let me know. A 28-year-elderly person said that she continued utilizing dating applications even though she had been abstinent for a long time, a reality she credited to despondency and low moxie: "I don't have a lot of tendency to date somebody."

"Sooner or later it just feels precisely equivalent to getting the hang of an air pocket popping game. I'm glad to be acceptable at it, however what am I truly accomplishing?" said an application client who depicted herself as abstinent by decision. Another lady composed that she was "excessively sluggish" to meet individuals, including: "I as a rule download dating applications on a Tuesday when I'm exhausted, sitting in front of the TV ... I don't make a decent attempt." Yet another lady said that she utilized an application, yet just "after two glasses of white wine—then I instantly erase it following two hours of unproductive swiping."

Numerous evaluates of web based dating, including a 2013 article by Dan Slater in The Atlantic, adjusted from his book A Million First Dates, have concentrated on the possibility that such a large number of alternatives can prompt "decision over-burden," which thusly prompts disappointment. Online daters, he contended, may be enticed to prop up back for encounters with new individuals; responsibility and marriage may endure. Michael Rosenfeld, a humanist who forces a longitudinal report to leave Stanford called "How Couples Meet and Stay Together," questions this theory; his exploration finds that couples who meet online will in general wed more rapidly than different couples, a reality that barely proposes uncertainty.

Possibly decision over-burden applies somewhat better than Slater envisioned. Possibly the issue isn't the individuals who date and date some more—they may even get hitched, if Rosenfeld is correct—however the individuals who are dismayed to such an extent that they don't make it off the love seat. This thought came up commonly in my discussions with individuals who depicted sex and dating lives that had gone into a profound freeze. Some utilized the term Catch 22 of decision; others alluded to alternative loss of motion (a term advanced by Black Mirror); still others summoned fobo ("dread of a superior choice").

But internet dating keeps on pulling in clients, to a limited extent because numerous individuals consider applications less distressing than the other options. Lisa Wade associates that graduates with secondary school or school hookup culture may respect the way that web based dating removes a portion of the vagueness from matching up (We've each selected in; I'm at any rate somewhat keen on you). The first run through my better half and I got together outside work, neither of us was certain whether it was a date. When you discover somebody by means of an application, there's less vulnerability.

As a 27-year-elderly person in Philadelphia put it: "I have frailties that make fun bar tease distressing. I don't care for the Is he into me? minute. I use dating applications because I need it to be evident this is a date and we are explicitly intrigued by each other. If it doesn't turn out, fine, yet there will never be an Is he requesting that I hang as a companion or as a date? feeling." Other individuals said they preferred the way that on an application, their first trades with an imminent date could play out by means of content as opposed to in an eye to eye or telephone discussion, which had.

In all dating markets, applications have all the earmarks of being generally useful to the exceptionally photogenic. As Emma, a 26-year-old virgin who sporadically attempts her karma with web based dating, sullenly let me know, "Dating applications make it simple for hot individuals—who as of now have the least demanding time." Christian Rudder, a prime supporter of OkCupid (one of the less appearance-driven dating administrations, in that it empowers point by point composed profiles), revealed in 2009 that the male clients who were evaluated most truly appealing by female clients got 11 fold the number of messages as the most reduced appraised men did; medium-evaluated men got around four fold the number of messages. The dissimilarity was starker for ladies: About 66% of messages went to the 33% of ladies who were evaluated most genuinely alluring. A later report by scientists at the University of Michigan and the Santa Fe Institute found that online daters of the two sexual orientations will in general seek after imminent mates who are on normal 25 percent more alluring than they are—probably not a triumphant system.

The very presence of web based dating makes it harder for anybody to make a suggestion face to face without appearing to be unseemly.

So where does this leave us? Numerous online daters invest a lot of energy seeking after individuals who are out of their association. Not many of their messages are returned, and significantly less lead to face to face contact. Best case scenario, the experience is able to puzzle (Why are for the most part these individuals swiping directly on me, then neglecting to finish?). Be that as it may, it can likewise be undermining, even difficult. Emma is, by her own portrayal, fat. She isn't embarrassed about her appearance, and intentionally incorporates a few full-body photographs in her dating profiles. By and by, men continue swiping directly on her profile just to insult her—when I talked with her, one person had as of late finished a content trade by sending her a gif of an overweight lady on a treadmill.

A significantly more serious issue might be the degree to which sentimental interest is presently being cordoned off into an anticipated, prearranged online setting, the very presence of which makes it harder for anybody, even those not utilizing the applications, to broaden a suggestion face to face without appearing to be wrong. What a hopeless stalemate.

4. Terrible Sex (Painfully Bad)

One particularly springlike morning in May, as Debby Herbenick and I strolled her child through a recreation center in Bloomington, Indiana, she shared a touch of guidance she now and again offers understudies at Indiana University, where she is a main sex specialist. "If you're with someone just because," she said equitably, "don't gag them, don't discharge all over, don't attempt to have butt-centric sex with them. These are everything that are only far-fetched to turn out well."

I'd searched out Herbenick to a limited extent because I was fascinated by an article she'd composed for The Washington Post suggesting that the sex decrease may have a silver covering. Herbenick had asked whether we may be seeing, in addition to other things, a retreat from coercive or in any case undesirable sex. Only a couple of decades prior, all things considered, conjugal assault was as yet legitimate in numerous states. As she pushed her little girl's carriage, she explained on the possibility that a portion of the sex downturn's causes could be a solid response to terrible sex—a subset of individuals "not engaging in sexual relations that they would prefer not to have any longer. Individuals feeling progressively engaged to state 'No thanks.' "

Bloomington is the informal capital of American sex investigate, a status that goes back to the 1940s, when the Indiana University scientist Alfred Kinsey's spearheading sex overviews initiated the field. It holds its standing on account of the efficiency of its researchers, and mostly to the scarcity of sex inquire about at different foundations. In 2009, Herbenick and her partners propelled the progressing National Survey of Sexual Health and Behavior, which is just the second broadly agent overview to analyze Americans' sexual experiences in detail—and the first to attempt to diagram them after some time. (The past national study, out of the University of Chicago, was directed only once, in 1992. Most other sex examine, including Kinsey's, has utilized what are known as accommodation tests, which don't speak to the populace on the loose. The long-running General Social Survey, which a lot of Jean Twenge's exploration depends on, is broadly delegate, however offers just a couple of conversation starters about sex.)

I asked Herbenick whether the NSSHB's discoveries gave her any hunches about what may have changed since the 1990s. She referenced the new ubiquity of sex toys, and a flood in hetero butt-centric sex. In 1992, the large University of Chicago review revealed that 20 percent of ladies in their late 20s had attempted butt-centric sex; in 2012, the NSSHB found a rate twice that. She likewise informed me regarding new information proposing that, contrasted and past ages, youngsters today are bound to take part in sexual practices predominant in pornography, similar to the ones she cautions her understudies against springing on an accomplice. The entirety of this may be frightening a few people away, she thought, and adding to the sex decrease.

"If you are a young lady," she included, looking down at her little girl, "and you're engaging in sexual relations and someone attempts to stifle you, I simply don't have the foggiest idea whether you'd need to return for all the more immediately."

A portion of herbenick's most calming research concerns the commonness of excruciating sex. In 2012, 30 percent of ladies said they'd encountered torment the last time they'd had vaginal intercourse; during butt-centric intercourse, 72 percent had. Regardless of whether these rates speak to an expansion (we have no reason for examination), they are troublingly high. Additionally, most ladies don't inform their accomplices regarding their agony. J. Dennis Fortenberry, the head of pre-adult medication at Indiana University's clinical school and a co-pioneer of the NSSHB, accepts that numerous young ladies and ladies have disguised that physical inconvenience goes with being female.

An especially distinctive outline of this originates from Lucia O'Sullivan, a University of New Brunswick brain science teacher who has distributed research archiving high paces of sexual brokenness among youths and youthful grown-ups. That work became out of a lunch quite a while back with a doctor from the college's understudy wellbeing focus, who disclosed to O'Sullivan that she was profoundly worried by all the vulvar gaps she and her associates were finding in their understudy patients. These ladies weren't revealing assault, yet the state of their privates indicated that they were suffering intercourse that was, truly, undesired. "They were engaging in sexual relations they didn't need, weren't stirred by," O'Sullivan says. The doctor revealed to her that the standard of care was to hand the ladies K-Y Jelly and send them out the door.

Difficult sex isn't new, yet there's motivation to imagine that pornography might be adding to some especially horrendous early sexual encounters. Studies show that, without top notch sex instruction, adolescent young men seek pornography for help getting sex—butt-centric sex and different acts ladies can discover excruciating are omnipresent in standard pornography. (It is not necessarily the case that butt-centric sex must be excruciating, yet rather that the variant most ladies are encountering is.) In a progression of top to bottom meetings, Cicely Marston of the London School of Hygiene and Tropical Medicine found that adolescent young men trying different things with butt-centric sex—maybe impacted by what they've found in pornography—may locate that unexpected, unlubricated infiltration is more difficult than it looks, and additionally anguishing for the beneficiary. A portion of her subjects seem to have compelled their accomplice; others appear to have depended on what another specialist depicted to me, clinically, as "nonconsensual substitution of butt-centric for vaginal sex."

In my meetings with young ladies, I heard an excessive number of cycles to tally of "he accomplished something I didn't care for that I later learned is a staple in pornography," gagging being one generally refered to model. Outside of pornography, a few people do make the most of what's known as sensual suffocation—they express limiting oxygen to the mind can make for increasingly extreme climaxes—yet it is hazardous and positions high on the rundown of things you shouldn't do to somebody except if asked to. Tess, a 31-year-elderly person in San Francisco, referenced that her previous hardly any sexual encounters had been with marginally more youthful men. "I've seen that they will in general go for gagging without earlier conversation," she said. Anna, the lady who depicted how dating applications could deflect cumbersomeness, revealed to me she'd been stifled so often that from the outset, she figured it was typical. "Many individuals don't understand you need to ask," she said.

As Marina Adshade, an educator at the University of British Columbia who examines the financial matters of sex and love, said to me, "Men have terrible sex and great sex. Be that as it may, when sex is awful for ladies, it's ridiculously awful. If ladies are staying away from sex, would they say they are attempting to keep away from the downright awful sex?"

Sex sets aside some effort to learn under the best of conditions, and these are not the best of conditions. Demonstrating your conduct after what you've seen on-screen can prompt what's known as "spectatoring"— that is, stressing over what you look like and sound while you're engaging in sexual relations, a conduct the sex analysts William H. Experts and Virginia E. Johnson sometime in the past set was terrible for sexual working. Some young ladies disclosed to me they felt constrained to copy pornography on-screen characters—and to accomplish climax from infiltration alone, which most ladies can't do. "It took me some time to be alright with the way that I don't need to be as vocal during sex as the young ladies appear to be in pornography," a 24-year-elderly person in Boston said. A 31-year-old in Phoenix clarified that as far as she can tell, pornography has caused men "to expect that they can make any lady climax by simply beating ceaselessly."

Learning sex with regards to one-off hookups isn't helping either.

5. Hindrance

"Twenty to thirty year olds don't care to get exposed—if you go to the rec center now, everybody under 30 will put their clothing on under the towel, which is a gigantic social shift," Jonah Disend, the organizer of the marking consultancy Redscout, revealed to Bloomberg a year ago. He said that plans for main room suites were advancing for a lot of a similar explanation: "They need their own changing rooms and restrooms, even in a couple." The article inferred that anyway "carefully impassive" Millennials may appear—an inference, possibly, to sexting—"they're pedantic face to face." Fitness offices the nation over are said to revamp storage spaces because of the requests of more youthful customers. "Old-clocks, folks that are 60 or more, have no issue with a group shower," one rec center originator revealed to The New York Times, including that Millennials require security.

A few spectators have recommended that another inconvenience with bareness may originate from the way that, by the mid-1990s, most secondary schools had quit expecting understudies to shower after exercise center class. Which bodes well—the less time you spend stripped, the less agreeable you are being bare. Be that as it may, individuals may likewise be recently stressed over what they resemble exposed. An enormous and developing assemblage of research reports that for the two people, web based life use is connected with body disappointment. What's more, a significant Dutch examination found that among men, recurrence of sex entertainment seeing was related with worry about penis size. I heard a lot of the equivalent from many men ("excessively bristly, not fit enough, not large enough regarding penis size," went one dismal reiteration). As indicated by examine by Debby Herbenick, how individuals feel about their privates predicts sexual working—and somewhere close to 20 and 25 percent of individuals, maybe impacted by pornography or plastic-medical procedure showcasing, feel contrarily. The matter of labiaplasty has gotten so worthwhile, she let me know in an email, "that you will really observe bulletins (indeed, announcements!) in certain urban areas publicizing it."

As one would envision, feeling great in your body is useful for your sexual coexistence. An audit of 57 examinations looking at the connection between ladies' self-perception and sexual conduct recommends that positive self-perception is connected to having better sex. On the other hand, not feeling great in your own skin confuses sex. If you don't need your accomplice to see you escaping the shower, how is oral sex going to function?

Possibly, for certain individuals, it isn't. The 2017 cycle of Match.com's Singles in America overview (co-drove by Helen Fisher and the Kinsey Institute's Justin Garcia) found that solitary Millennials were 66 percent more outlandish than individuals from more seasoned ages to appreciate accepting oral sex. Which doesn't bode especially well for female joy: Among banded together sex acts, cunnilingus is probably the surest ways for ladies to have climaxes.

Ian Kerner, the New York sex specialist, disclosed to me that he works with a great deal of men who might want to perform oral sex however are rebuked by their accomplice. "I realize the generalization is often that men are the ones who would prefer not to perform it, however I locate the turn around," he said. "A great deal of ladies will say when I'm talking to them secretly, 'I just can hardly imagine how a person needs to be down there, likes to do that. It's the ugliest piece of my body.' " When I got some information about oral sex, an entirely sizable minority of ladies sounded a comparable note. "Getting makes me apprehensive. It feels more private than entrance," kept in touch with one lady. "I become so unsure and think that its difficult to appreciate," composed another.

Over the previous 20 years, the way sex scientists consider want and excitement has expanded from an at first limited spotlight on boost to one that considers restraint to be similarly, if not progressively, significant. (The term restraint, for these reasons, implies whatever meddles with or forestalls excitement, extending from poor mental self-view to distractedness.) In her book Come as You May be, Emily Nagoski, who prepared at the Kinsey Institute, thinks about the cerebrum's fervor framework to the gas pedal in a vehicle, and its hindrance framework to the brakes. The principal turns you on; the second turns you off. For some, individuals, inquire about proposes, the brakes are more delicate than the quickening agent.

That mood killers matter more than turn-ons may sound commonsensical, however truth be told, this knowledge is inconsistent with most well-known perspectives on sexual issues. When individuals talk about tending to an absence of want, they will in general spotlight on fuel, or incitement—erotica, Viagra, the K-Y Jelly they were distributing at the New Brunswick understudy wellbeing focus. These things are useful to numerous individuals by and large, yet they won't make you need to have intercourse if your brakes are completely locked in.

In my meetings, hindrance appeared to be a consistent ally to numerous individuals who'd been abstinent for quite a while. The majority of them portrayed forbearance not as something they had grasped (because of strict conviction, state) to such an extent as something they'd wound up sponsored into because of injury, uneasiness, or discouragement. Dispiritingly however obviously, rape was summoned by numerous individuals of the ladies who said they'd quit sex. The other two variables come as no extraordinary stun either: Rates of uneasiness and wretchedness have been ascending among Americans throughout recent decades, and by certain records have risen strongly generally among individuals in their adolescents and 20s. Uneasiness stifles want for a great many people. What's more, in an especially terrible catch-22, both wretchedness and the antidepressants used to treat it can likewise diminish want.

"I have an advisor and this is one of the fundamental things we're dealing with," a 28-year-elderly person I'll call April kept in touch with me, by method for clarifying that, inferable from serious nervousness, she'd never laid down with anybody or been seeing someone. "I've had a couple of kisses and gone to a respectable halfway point (as the children state) and it truly has never been beneficial for me." When we later talked by telephone, she disclosed to me that in youth, she'd been timid, overweight, and "extremely, scared of young men." April isn't abiogenetic (she expresses gratefulness for her Magic Bullet vibrator). She's simply terrified of closeness. Every now and then she goes on dates with men she meets through her activity in the book business or on an application, however when things get physical, she freezes. "I leaped out of somebody's vehicle once to evade him kissing me," she said pitiably. As we were finishing the discussion, she referenced to me a story by the British essayist Helen Oyeyemi, which depicts a writer of romance books who is covertly a virgin. "She doesn't have anybody, and she's simply stuck. It's sort of a fantasy—she lives in the garret of an enormous, old house, composing these sentimental stories again and again, yet nothing ever occurs for her. I consider her constantly."

In trades like these, I was struck by what an incapacitating and endless loop despondency and forbearance can be. The information show that engaging in sexual relations makes individuals more joyful (to a limited extent, in any event; for those seeing someone, more than once seven days doesn't appear to bring an extra satisfaction knock). However despondency represses want, in the process denying individuals who are famished of satisfaction one of its latent capacity sources. Are increasing paces of misery adding to the sex downturn? More likely than not. Be that as it may, mightn't a decrease in sex and closeness additionally be prompting despondency?

In addition, what examine we have on explicitly latent grown-ups recommends that, for the individuals who want a sexual coexistence, there might be such a mind-bending concept as standing by excessively long. Among individuals who are explicitly unpracticed at age 18, around 80 percent will turn out to be explicitly dynamic when they are 25. However, the individuals who haven't increased sexual experience by their mid-20s are considerably less liable to ever do as such. The creators of a recent report in The Journal of Sexual Medicine conjectured that "if a man or lady has not had sex by age 25, there is a sensible possibility [he or she] will stay a virgin at any rate until age 45." Research by Stanford's Michael Rosenfeld affirms that, in adulthood, genuine singledom is an unquestionably more steady classification than the vast majority of us have envisioned. Throughout a year, he reports, just 50 percent of hetero single ladies in their 20s go on any dates—and more established ladies are even less inclined to do as such.

Different wellsprings of sexual hindrance talk unmistakably to the manner in which we live today. For instance, lack of sleep unequivocally smothers want—and rest quality is risked at this point regular practices like checking one's telephone medium-term. (For ladies, getting an additional hour of rest predicts a 14 percent more noteworthy probability of engaging in sexual relations the following day.) In her new book, Better Sex Through Mindfulness, Lori Brotto, an obstetrics-and-gynecology educator at the University of British Columbia, audits lab inquire about indicating that foundation interruption of the sort we're all swimming in now moreover hoses excitement, in the two people.

In what manner can such easily overlooked details—a terrible night's rest, poor quality interruption—rout something as basic as sex? One answer, which I got notification from a couple of quarters, is that our sexual cravings are intended to be effectively stifled. Humanity needs sex, however singular people don't.

Among the logical inconsistencies within recent memory is this: We live in uncommon physical security, but then something about present day life, extremely late current life, has activated in a large number of us autonomic reactions related with risk—tension, consistent filtering of our environment, erratic rest. Under these conditions, endurance bests want. As Emily Nagoski likes to call attention to, no one ever kicked the bucket of sexlessness: "We can starve to death, bite the dust of drying out, even bite the dust of lack of sleep. Be that as it may, no one ever passed on of not having the option to get laid."

WHY DIRTY TALK

Harder. Continue onward, don't stop. Better believe it, you like that, infant?

As constrained as it sounds when you read it, a large number of us love hearing dirty talk in the room. We lose ourselves in the warmth of enthusiasm and take on a persona that turns us on in the most devious, eccentric ways. In any case, there's a whole other world to it than that. What is it about sensual correspondence that builds our sexual excitement? When we look past the unusualness, we may locate there's a whole other world to dirty talk than our craving to draw out our wild side.

1. Sex On The Brain

It starts in the brain.

The mind is viewed as a more remarkable sexual organ than even male and female genitalia because it's the place sex drive comes from. The perfect measure of dirty talk will energize the psyche. Be that as it may, there is a difference in how every sexual orientation's limbic framework functions in the cerebrum.

Two regions in the nerve center, the preoptic territory and the superchiasmatic core, have unmistakable capacities in female and male cerebrums, as per an examination distributed in the diary Hormone Research. The preoptic zone, engaged with mating conduct, is more than multiple times bigger in men than ladies and contains multiple times more cells. In the mean time, the superchiasmatic core, engaged with circadian rhythms and propagation cycles differs fit as a fiddle: Males have a core that is formed like a circle, while ladies have a greater amount of an extended one.

A bigger nerve center for men implies all the more flowing testosterone to invigorate the craving for sex. A lower testosterone level and a littler nerve center in ladies, then again, implies their sex drive isn't as solid as a man's. These organic differences are only the numerous ways people cerebrum work differs when it comes to sex.

Daryl Cioffi, having some expertise in couples, connections, sex, neuropsychology, and proprietor of Polaris Counseling and Consulting in Patucket, R.I., says dirty talk is an entire brain and body understanding.

"Individuals particularly appreciate dirty talking because it enacts all areas of your mind while your body is additionally getting invigorated," Cioffi revealed to Medical Daily. "Comparative zones of the cerebrum are addressed during dirty talk as when we revile. In this way, all the time through your's eyes, the dirtier the better."

For instance, numerous influential ladies in their regular daily existences and occupations appreciate being increasingly accommodating in the bed, says Cioffi, because it invigorates the amygdala. This cerebrum area is our dread community that is vigorously associated with energy and delight during sex. The murmurs, groans, and shouts joined by dirty talk are totally prepared by the cerebrum's hearing place, including the worldly flap, the frontal projection, and the occipital projection.

All things considered, the psyche is an erogenous zone. The cerebrum and how it sorts out the remainder of our erogenous zones is additional proof of the urgent job of the mind in deciding both sex drive and sexual joy.

Asking what our accomplices need from us and what we need from them opens up the lines of correspondence to show we're available to switching things up in the room. Verbalizing the sexual jobs we need and hearing what our accomplices need to do to us is fundamental in sexual excitement.

As indicated by Dr. Ava Cadell, proficient speaker, essayist, and sex advisor in Los Angeles, Calif., couples take part in dirty talk to "uplift their excitement and offer dreams that they might not have any desire to transform into the real world, yet talking about them can be shockingly better."

2. Imparting Sexual Fantasies In The Bedroom

Submitting sexual acts and talking dirty include two totally different attitudes. Dirty talk is something we do without anyone else, instead of physical sex acts. This suggestive discourse, therefore, serves to release the enthusiasm for new sexual acts that may not for the most part be of intrigue.

"People can get settled and acquainted with utilizing expressions and language and depictions that express their needs and needs," Dr. Fran Walfish, Beverly Hills psychotherapist, creator of The Self-Aware Parent, and master specialist on WE TV's Sex Box revealed to Medical Daily. "Work on communicating your requirements and needs and urge your accomplice to do likewise and be prepared to convey the merchandise."

A recent report distributed in the Journal of Social and Personal Relationships found the more agreeable we are talking about sex, the more good our sexual experiences will turn into. As indicated by the analysts, even the smallest nervousness about correspondence influenced whether accomplices were imparting or not. It likewise legitimately influenced their fulfillment. The individuals who communicated during sex were bound to encounter sexual fulfillment. At the end of the day, participating in an exchange that feels great with our accomplice can increase the sexual experience.

April Masini, relationship master and creator, revealed to Medical Daily: "Talking dirty can upgrade sex because it's another layer of sexual conduct past physical sexual acts."

Dirty talk can likewise excite accomplices to the point of climax. A few ladies and men can really get so turned on by dirty talk that they will get wet or hard and climax, even without genital incitement. Masini says, the intensity of dirty talk can permit somebody to get "out of their own head" and into the state of mind.

3. Dirty Talk And The 'Great Girl' Complex

The "great young lady" unpredictable, like the Madonna-Whore complex, is only one feature of what men need. Sex consistently is by all accounts the line that the "great young lady" crosses where they simply need to sink somebody request to be viewed as a "trouble maker." Pop culture has sustained this complex from melodies as thicke Robin's "Obscured Lines" where he "knows" she needs it because she's a creature and it's in her temperament, to Usher's "No doubt!" where Ludacris recognizes "we" (the men) need a woman in the road and oddity in the bed.

Dirty talk is a freeing experience for ladies to separate this outlook and become agreeable in their sexuality and wants. It's the place individuals welcome their dreams and where that no nonsense adaptation of an individual will appreciate being tied up, being called specific sorts of names, and utilizing dirty words for genital parts when else they wouldn't consider such conduct, says Walfish.

It brings down hindrances and uncovers room characters by permitting accomplices to go a layer further inside our ordinary selves.

For instance, a few ladies may get turned on by words like "skank" or "prostitute," despite the fact that they think that its hostile outside the room. Ladies can assume responsibility for the word and use it on their own terms. This phonetic trade can uncover the darker dreams of the mind and be happened in the protection of the room.

A lady who calls up her accomplice grinding away to state to him "when you return home darling, I'm going to let you attach me to the bedpost, bind me, and capture me," says Walfish, is vocalizing her dream outside the room.

"One chance is possibly she has a needy character and perhaps she loves submitting to a prevailing, incredible power," she said. "Or then again perhaps she fantasizes about being the predominant one and is reluctant to put that on to her person to do it first, so she tries things out."

Fundamentally, when we expect a persona through dirty talk or pretending, we have a simpler time being sexual.

4. Dirty Talk And Intimacy

Dirty talk gives individuals authorization to give up to their most profound, darkest, most stunning dreams. Sex should be dirty, sexual, and above all good times.

Sexuality makes closeness for a couple and turns into the paste of the relationship. Great sex is an indicator of a decent relationship.

"Sex isn't only a physical discharge or a declaration of adoration and love. It's a method to work things out and process injuries, of all shapes and sizes," Masini said.

Dirty talk isn't for debases, it's tied in with upgrading your sexual experience and vocalizing your sexual needs. More men need ladies to do it, as per Cadell, and that is the reason ladies do it, to satisfy their men. "Ladies are increasingly sound-related and men are progressively visual," she said.

For dirty talk to be fruitful, it must be one good turn deserves another. The two individuals ought to do it so there's no kind of enmity or hatred or force battle.

It's everything about fill in the clear. "I love it when you clear me," or "Your clear is so hot."

All things considered, says Masini, "talking dirty is simply sexual introduction. It's everything about the sex."

I didn't think I'd be into dirty talk before I attempted it. I'm a tremendous aficionado of exactness, and I wouldn't consider somebody my "daddy" except if they really were. Be that as it may, the first run through a man did the unimaginable and began saying words to me during sex (hot words, not "hello can you scooch over" or my run of the mill exhibition), I ended up strangely turned on. I pondered about the brain research behind dirty talk and why it turns individuals on to make statements in the room (or vehicle or washroom or any place you like to have intercourse) they wouldn't state in any case.

One explanation individuals may appreciate dirty talk is because sex is a destresser, so they might be less reluctant about saying what they're really doing and feeling. As indicated by a recent report done by the National Center for Biotechnology Information, having a climax discharges oxytocin, which is a synthetic that decreases your feelings of anxiety. Bringing down your feelings of anxiety implies you're likely not so much restrained but rather more liable to state precisely what you need or think, regardless of whether you ordinarily wouldn't in your regular daily existences. Possibly you have something truly dirty to state about your accomplice's body, however you'd act naturally cognizant saying that for any assortment of reasons, but then, it sneaks out right at the peak. If you have something extremely dirty on the tip of your tongue, it might be bound to turn out as you're accomplishing climax.

Dirty talk enacts our cerebrums, which is really where a ton of the incitement from sex originates from. You may have heard the expression "thinking with your lower head" (spoiler alert: They mean penis), however, your upper head is doing a great deal of the work. It's not simply privates that are liable for sexual incitement, in spite of the fact that your sexual organs are significant also. The job the cerebrums play in sexual delight could clarify why you probably won't be in the temperament for sex if you're despondent or worried for different reasons, as indicated by an investigation in Hormone Research in 2005, two pieces of the nerve center — the preoptic territory and the suprachiasmatic core — are liable for sexual joy. Dirty talk animates them two, which prepares individuals to go explicitly. As per Cosmopolitan, groaning or murmuring during sex discharging a neurochemical response that turns the two gatherings on. So if you're turned on by words during sex, there could be a valid justification why.

A few people appreciate the accommodation of dirty talk, especially if they have incredible jobs in their everyday lives. As indicated by Medical Daily, dirty talk animates the amygdala, which is the dread focus of the cerebrum and controls energy and delight. Similar vibes that cause individuals appreciate obligation additionally lead individuals to feel stimulated by accommodation, as indicated by American Dating Society. So also, dirty talk causes the dirty-talker to seem certain, so it very well may be a job inversion if one individual is increasingly sure about their regular day to day existences. Not every person is turned on by dirty talk that causes them to feel like a compliant, however, so make a point to talk to your accomplice before attempting it.

Dirty talk can really improve your sexual coexistence regardless of whether you use it outside the room. As indicated by a 2011 Psychology Today report, embeddings little, provocative expressions into your discussion with your accomplice during the day can prompt better sex. It very well may be as basic as murmuring "I need to whittle down that succulent tomato" while holding a tomato (which is really a usually articulated expression for me in any organization). If saying something dirty outside the room makes you reluctant, you're unquestionably not the only one, and you can in any case get turned on by dirty talk in the room. No one can really tell where you will be caught, yet that can be a piece of the good times. Along these lines, if you consider talking dirty outside the room provocative, check out it (and taste the tomato, it's tasty). If you need to attempt it however you're anxious, consider carrying it up with your accomplice previously to ensure they'll be open — their energize could assist you with building certainty to state something edgier in broad daylight.

There are numerous mental and neurological reasons why we appreciate dirty talk. I didn't open my mouth during sex until I was around 23 (and indeed, I imply that precisely how it sounds), however once I did, I understood I truly preferred it. Presently I get why – my mind has been wired to look for delight. There are a wide range of substance responses going on in my mind during sex, and dirty talk can enhance a large number of them. Additionally, I love talking – who doesn't?

There are not many lines in music that bring me as much happiness as, "Pussy so great I got her a pet," from the splendid expressive brain of Jason Derulo. The sex was extraordinary; here's a parakeet. Reason me, Jason?! No lady needs to consider pet consideration while engaging in sexual relations. While the tune should be a tribute to talking dirty, start to finish it's all out strange. At a certain point he requests that a lady "suck my penis," which couldn't be to a lesser degree a provocative method to start a sensual caress.

However, I can't accuse Jason Derulo. Or if nothing else not Jason Derulo alone. Regardless, ladies have had magazine upon magazine (and boundless pornography recordings) show us how to sound attractive in bed, and goodness gracious do we comprehend its estimation. In the interim, it's splendidly satisfactory for men to be quiet the whole time they're engaging in sexual relations, yet that shouldn't be the situation. You'll likely suck at dirty talk in the first place, however nobody at any point improved at something without a little practice. What's more, it will be justified, despite all the trouble; next to no is more sultry than very much done dirty talk. That is the reason ladies will in general expend increasingly composed pornography; it's a huge piece of why 50 Shade of Gray progressed admirably. Ladies truly like dirty talk! Also, the vast majority of them aren't getting quite a bit of it.

I get it, however. It tends to be difficult to vocalize during sex without seeming like a darn blockhead. In a tweet I will recall perpetually, a companion of mine portrayed the most lamentable dirty talk he'd at any point done, in which he really told a lady "I'm going to screw your moronic pussy." I know! Out of consideration for sex havers all over, I'm going to spread out how to talk dirty such that will take sex with your accomplice to the following level.

You will sound moronic (get over yourself).

As a matter of first importance, likewise with everything identified with sex, you need to submit to the way that dirty talk is dubiously ludicrous. Sex is fundamentally simply scouring (at least two) exposed bodies together because it feels better, so normally any portrayal of the demonstration is somewhat senseless. You need to surrender to this, much like you surrender to the possibility of someone else seeing you bare. Push through the ponderousness. It might appear to be weird, however take a stab at expressing dirty things when you're absolutely alone as training. On the drive to work simply state, "I need to screw you so awful" at a typical volume until it doesn't cause you to recoil. We're every one of the a piece explicitly subdued right now, it requires some push to fix that. Odds are, at some point, you'll state something extraordinarily idiotic, and that is fine. Keep it moving. Or on the other hand stop and chuckle with your accomplice. Either is hot and fun.

Utilize the fitting wording.

This ought to be self-evident, yet if Jason Derulo's verses are any sign, it isn't. Some portion of not sounding crazy is utilizing provocative terms for body parts. You aren't in a specialist's office. Kindly don't consider your dick your penis. It would be ideal if you Likewise for vagina. Tits and boobs are both satisfactory, yet don't you dare utilize the c-word (except if your accomplice has asked you expressly to do as such). There's no compelling reason to get extravagant or idyllic; you're not composing an article for AP Lit, alright? Adhere to the works of art. They work which is as it should be. Cockerel and pussy are acceptable, acceptably dirty spots to begin. They're forbidden enough that you wouldn't state them around your chief, but at the same time they're not insolent or clinical, which is actually the tone you ought to be going for.

Mention to me what you need what you super need.

There's a minute in 27 Dresses (if it's not too much trouble don't hesitate to cook me for my horrendous preference for motion pictures) where Katherine Heigl affirms her affection for James Marsden and afterward he says, provocatively, "get here." Which resembles the most sizzling thing ever. (Look at this clasp at 1:36 if you're confounded). Practically any blend of come/get here will do. It accomplishes crafted by dirty talk without saying anything express or grimy. At the end of the day, it's an incredible spot to begin if you're new to the entire dirty talk thing. When your accomplice is in reality near you, you can catch up with something like "I've been contemplating this throughout the day," or "God, I need to screw you so gravely." Anything that plainly communicates your longing is perfect dirty talk. We often consider men being too open (read: unpleasant) about needing ladies explicitly—taking a gander at you, catcallers—yet when it comes to suitably and consciously telling your accomplice you need to blast, men sort of suck at it. Here's a simple guide: Don't be reluctant to inform somebody you're unmistakably concerning to have intercourse with the amount you need to engage in sexual relations with them. That is hot. OK? Great.

Direness is hot.

Similarly, telling somebody that you don't simply need them, you need them right presently is hot. You clearly need to regard that because you need somebody currently, doesn't mean they have to engage in sexual relations with you right away. In any case, when you're there, "I need you at this moment," works truly well. Don't hesitate to depict the thing you really need to do. "I gotta go down on you at the present time." obviously, this isn't you saying what you will do paying little heed to your accomplice's assent; it resembles utilizing your signal—it's a marker of what you intend to do straightaway. It gives a (hot) window for your accomplice to state, "Pause, play with my boobs first before you do that," or whatever else they may need.

I like it like that.

An entirely underestimated procedure of dirty talk is just saying what you like. "It feels so great when you X my Y," is simple, dirty, and hot. Right now, engaging in sexual relations with somebody is one of only a handful not many occasions it's absolutely worthy to remark on their body (in a positive, adoring way!). Think, "Your tits are great, I need to _____ them," or "You look so hot when you _____." Dirty talk shouldn't be only vile; it tends to be loving as well.

Try not to guide somebody until you know it's cool.

Newsflash: not every person needs to have similar sorts of sex. In this way, the way in to the hottest dirty talk is to speak with your accomplice enough to recognize what makes them go. You don't must have a long, plunk down talk, yet you should see whether your accomplice likes being determined what to do before being immediate with them. "Suck my chicken," or something likewise vuglar which could without much of a stretch put an end to an in any case fun time if you express it to an inappropriate individual. Sooner or later when you're not in sex, you can ask, "Hello, do you like being determined what to do in bed, or is that a side road?" Make it clear you regard that they aren't required to play out any demonstration essentially because you said to. I guarantee you—guarantee—any accomplice you have will be excited that you talked to them about sex in a sound, open way.

Dirty talk is a piece of the dream of sex, and dream doesn't generally make an interpretation of flawlessly to the real world. If you tell somebody, "Flip over the present moment," and they react with, "No, I like this position," is fine! Try not to close down, or feel like you messed up. Dirty talk is only there to increase the fervor and help you convey what you need. You should, obviously, additionally be asking what your accomplice needs, yet there's little more smoking than a person who's not humiliated to request what he needs in bed.

DIRTY TALK GUIDELINES, HOW TO SAY THE RIGHT THINGS AND PHRASES TO GET YOU STARTED

Does the idea of your accomplice saying, "talk dirty to me" send you into a frenzy? You're not the only one if the possibility of dirty talk (past "yes" and various groans) causes you to feel cumbersome.

Here's some uplifting news to ease the heat off: When it comes to sounding sultry, ladies can without much of a stretch sex-up the sound of their voice, while men essentially can't, as per an Albright College study. (Truth be told, folks were really observed as less appealing when they attempted to sound attractive.) If your accomplice is a lady, then congratulations: Your lesbian dirty talk is going to be hot as hellfire.

The drawback? Because you have a characteristic oral capacity (hi, rough room voice!) doesn't mean you realize which words will put you both in the state of mind. "Numerous individuals feel senseless talking dirty," says Jaiya, a sex instructor and creator of Blow Each Other Away. "Because they don't have the foggiest idea what to state, they get entangled."

Be that as it may, when you do realize what to state? The sexual result is tremendous. That is the reason we've assembled a couple of essential rules on the most proficient method to talk dirty to assist you with taking advantage of your inward sex goddess. Get ready to excite your accomplice more than ever with your mouth.

Do: Discover Their Trigger Words

Odds are, your accomplice has a specific most loved term for their body parts-just as for sexual acts, similar to intercourse and oral-that turn them on the most. Jaiya calls these trigger words, since the insignificant sound of them is often enough to wrench up his excitement. "Start by sending dirty instant messages to and fro," proposes Ruth Neustifter, Ph.D., creator of The Nice Girl's Guide to Talking Dirty. "This is an incredible method to make sense of what words they like." Your line: "I can hardly wait to see you today around evening time. Reveal to me all the spots you need me to contact you." They'll utilize the words they find generally sexual, helping you make your room vocab.

Do: Update Them on Your Arousal

"I'm so wet at the present time." "I'm going to come." "You feel mind blowing." These minute by-minute updates assist you with tuning into your own excitement an often-difficult undertaking for us-while giving him a suggestive earful. "When you talk about what's going on in your own body, you're carrying attention to it," says Jaiya. "In addition, you're stimulating them considerably more, because they'rethinking, 'Yes! I'm turning her on.' That causes them to feel progressively sure." We call that a success win. (Related: How to Have an Orgasm Every Time)

Try not to: Feel Pressure

"Dirty talk" is maybe a misnomer, because room chitchat doesn't need to be unrefined to be a turn-on. "A few people see reviling as totally un-exciting," says Neustifter. "The words that turn your accomplice on may be delicate and cherishing that can be similarly as exceptionally stirring," Jaiya includes. If you don't know which they like, take a stab at substituting sweet expressions (for example "I love it when you kiss me") with more scandalous ones (for example "I need your [body part] inside me"), and see what fires up them the most.

Do: Stick with What Works for You

"Ladies believe they should seem like pornography stars," says Yvonne Fulbright, Ph.D., creator of Sultry Sex Talk to Seduce Any Lover. In any case, because Jenna Jameson said it doesn't mean you have to-the most blazing words are the ones that get you in the zone, regardless of whether they're similarly agreeable. "If you're not being authentic or you aren't happy, they'll will feel that," says Jaiya.

What's more, you don't need to utilize a profound, throaty voice. "Your tone can be interesting and kidding. It tends to be adorable or prodding, guiltless, or totally underhanded," says Neustifter. "I urge ladies to consider times when they feel the most certain and lighthearted." If you feel your best giving introductions busy working, for instance, an incredible room vibe might be your go-to; if you love snickering with your companions, an enjoyment approach might be better. (Additionally important: Spend time jerking off to make sense of what you like.)

Do: Master the Art of One-Word Dirty Talk

Attempting to string together a full, dingy sentence can really pack down your longing, since you're inside your head, says Jaiya. "When I do sexuality workshops, the word 'yes' is reliably one of individuals' preferred words," says Neustifter. Other hot words that can remain solitary: "quicker," "harder," and "increasingly." One-word orders let them realize they're working superbly, says Jaiya. They're what might be compared to a groan.

Try not to: Focus Too Much on Size

If you're dating a man, know this: Sure, some folks love being told their penis is amazing, however for other people, catching wind of size may help them to remember their own weaknesses, says Neustifter. A superior course: Talk about how firm his erection is. "By and large, individuals react well to hearing how stirred their private parts are," she says.

Do: Outline Their Qualities That Excite You

Talking about specific sexual acts can be uber-scaring particularly when you're first making sense of how to talk dirty. "It's oftentimes simpler to talk about traits or articles how attractive a bit of clothing is, or that you truly like his facial hair stubble," says Neustifter. So start with illustrative proclamations of what turns you on about your accomplice. A great many people like to be commended. Additionally, it's practically difficult to tumble when you're telling somebody how much their body energizes you.

Do: Tell Them What You're Going to Do

Prepared for cutting edge dirty talk? Educate your accomplice concerning the hot moves you need to perform. "It's simpler for ladies to mind take than to state, 'This is what I need you to do,'" says Jaiya. So slide into it by recommending a move you've attempted in the past that both of you delighted in. (Like, for instance, these sex positions for clit incitement.) That way, you realize they'll get your recommendation decidedly, which can cause you to feel progressively certain assuming responsibility.

It's a territory of sex that causes many individuals to feel senseless because they're uncertain of how to go about it without feeling absurd.

When somebody says "Talk dirty to me infant... " in the room the ideally destined to-be dirty talker in a split second freezes like a splashing wet move of tissue being tossed out of an igloo in Antartica.

What would it be advisable for you to state? What do they need you to state? Consider the possibility that you state excessively. Consider the possibility that you state pretty much nothing.

Dirty talk, much the same as sex itself, is something that should be aligned to the person that is hearing the dirty talk from their accomplice.

Possibly something that you qualify as dirty talk is hostile, or funny, or crazy to your accomplice.

This is a definitive manual for dirty talk, strolling you through the things to for the most part maintain a strategic distance from, incorporate, and avoid by and large with the goal for you to overwhelm the universe of dirty talk.

(For the record, I don't put stock in the words "dirty talk" since there's nothing dirty about sex or talking about sex. Oh dear, this is the thing that individuals call it so I need to meet society where it's at present at.)

Five General Dirty Talk Guidelines

I'll get into specific expressions you can utilize immediately, on the whole, a few rules to assist you with getting your dark belt from the dirty talk dojo.

1) Before Sex, Say What You Want – During Sex, Say What You Like

A decent general guideline with dirty talk is to mention to your accomplice what you need to do to them/with them before you're doing it, and afterward while you're doing it, mention to them what you're loving about it.

For instance, possibly your accomplice has a moderately high sex drive however their motor possibly gets fired up when they're pondering sex. They need to engage in sexual relations all the more often yet it simply doesn't enter their thoughts all that often. The arrangement? Dirty talk.

Once more, this will all be founded on what you authentically want right now, however saying something along the lines of "I'm attempting to complete work yet I can't quit pondering a week ago when we were 69'ing and your scrumptious juices were streaming into my mouth" could be what pushes them over the edge to bouncing you.

Any announcement about what you have enjoyed doing with them, or that you are imagining doing with them, is an extraordinary method to slip into a super-vocal sex meeting.

And keeping in mind that you're wasting time, giving your accomplice continuous input about what you're appreciating is an incredible method to urge them to give you a greater amount of that thing, and furthermore gives your sexual play the additional edge of getting to a greater extent a multi-tactile encounter.

2) Be Descriptive

For many individuals, it's the subtleties of dirty talk that make it such a large amount of a turn on.

For the record, there's literally nothing amiss with explanations like "Better believe it, I like that," "You look so hot at this moment," and "I love engaging in sexual relations with you."

In any case, they can be supercharged in an enormous way if you shift them each with a touch of expressive detail.

"No doubt, I like that" becomes "Gracious my god, continue doing that. I love your enormous/little hands all over my rear end/balls/chest/and so forth.. You are the hottest individual on earth."

"You look so hot at the present time" transforms into "You are superior to anything any dream I would ever thought of. I screwing love you and your ideal/delightful/provocative enormous/little (body part)."

I love engaging in sexual relations with you" changes into "I love it when you snatch the sheets when you're going to come. I love the wonderful way your breath stops when I put my mouth on your (embed accomplice's favored name for their privates here). There's no place else I'd preferably be over within you/over you at this moment."

Presently... isn't that better??

3) Use All Of Your Senses

Probably the quickest approaches to help the force and sexual, drawing in nature of your dirty talk is to begin utilizing multi-tactile unmistakable words.

The vast majority dirty talk with two of their essential detects: sight and contact (for example "You look so hot/You feel so great").

While there's nothing amiss with adhering to your customary range of familiarity by remaining inside the parameters of these two predominant sexual faculties, there's such a great amount of enjoyable to be had by letting your graphic creative mind go out of control.

– I love the wonderful way you taste/smell. I could become inebriated off of your juices/fragrance.

– I love the sounds you make

– You sound so hot when I'm going down on you

– I need to screw you until I feel that sweet minimal pussy grasping around my chicken

– I need you to cum so hard that I feel your cockerel beating within me.

DIRTY TALK EXAMPLES

Dirty talk isn't for everybody. It is difficult for everybody to communicate, in words and for all to hear, what they need to do to their accomplice or what they need their accomplice to do to them. Some adoration it, some detest it, and some fair can't figure out how to pull it off without snickering. What's more, there can likewise be the battle of word decision when you're evaluating dirty talk.

"Dirty talk is about the subtleties," sex teacher, Lola Jean, tells Bustle. "We need to paint an image with our words so in all actuality, falling back on a specific notice of sexual orientation and privates is *kind of* sluggish. Consider dirty talk likewise as prodding, you can decide to paint a whole picture for somebody or let them fill in the lines with their own creative mind. It relies upon the level which you definitely know the individual and their requirement for self-sufficiency."

Obviously, not every person is into something very similar or requirements to hear something very similar so as to be stirred. That is certainly something to think about.

"I like giving individuals choices which both permits me to become familiar with them and furthermore lets them control a specific bit too," Lola Jean says. "It resembles a provocative pick your own experience. Additionally this is a brilliant area to investigate different things you might be awkward with... Cause an emphasis on what you to can include, to make you more quiet versus what you remove."

Here are 11 instances of talking dirty that have nothing at all to do with sexual orientation.

1. "I'm Taking Off Your Clothes, Do I..."

Have a go at giving your accomplice choices to choose what they need straightaway. It's a "pick your own experience," as Lola Jean calls it.

For instance, if you return home and are going to have intercourse, you can ask your accomplice what they need. Would they like to be prodded for somewhat first? Do they need you to gradually take off their garments, each catch in turn, possibly with your mouth? Or on the other hand do they need you to tear their garments, hop on top, and go straight for it?

When you give your accomplice choices with your dirty talk, you not just permit them to assume a functioning job, however it additionally causes you comprehend what your accomplice likes and what gets them off.

2. "Before I Kiss You, I Hold The Back Of Your Neck, Do You Say..."

Once more, choices are everything, particularly in the learning procedure. Lola Jeans proposes offering these four decisions:

"If you don't mind

"Make me."

"I need you."

"You better procure it."

Every one has a different opinion, contingent upon the dynamic of your relationship.

3. "We're Going On A Date Tonight, What Turns You On More?"

Obviously better than pre-gaming with liquor for a date, is pre-gaming with dirty talk far before you even interact with one another.

Lola Jean proposes giving your accomplice an in depth of how you're preparing by means of content and leaving them alone piece of the procedure. Here are four alternatives to give your accomplice if you're new to talking dirty, as indicated by Lola Jean.

"I reveal to you a procedure about my preparing, sending you pictures."

"You find a workable pace outfit and clothing alternatives."

"I mention to you what I will do when we meet."

"I send you a playlist to tune in to before our date."

4. "I'm Thinking About The Last Time I Saw You And My Body Is Aching For The Next."

When you message your accomplice, "I'm contemplating the last time I saw you and my body is throbbing for the following," you're complimenting them, something everybody adores, except you're communicating your craving for them, an overwhelming inclination for them — something a few people may state is more delectable than bootlicking.

5. "The Only Thing That I Crave More Than Your Body Is Your Mind."

Truly need to get your accomplice worked up with some dirty talk? Then remember to address their brain: "The main thing that I want more than your body is your psyche."

Sexuality is more about what's in your mind than what's between your legs all things considered.

6. "Think About The Place You Like Most Where I Touch You. Presently Let Your Mind Wander And Show Me The Way."

When you're talking dirty, it shouldn't be an uneven discussion. If it is, then things are rattled. While you're under no commitment to talk dirty if you're not happy with it, then you can at any rate give bearings with your hands.

For instance, if your accomplice says to you, "Think about the spot you like most where I contact you. Presently let your brain meander and show me the way," you can react without saying word. On the other side, if you realize your accomplice isn't open to talking dirty, this is additionally an incredible line because it permits them to be included, while saying nothing, keeping them in their usual range of familiarity.

7. "Simply Thinking Of The Way Your Skin Reacts To My Touch Is Enough To Send Shivers Down My Own Spine."

Take a stab at saying, "Simply thinking about the manner in which your skin responds to my touch is sufficient to send shudders down my own spine."

8. "I'm Thinking About The Next Time I'll See You And Have A Urge To..."

You may need your accomplice to realize that you're so stirred by them, in any event, when they're nowhere to be found, that the inclination to drop all that you're doing and go to them presently is genuine. For instance have a go at saying, "I'm pondering whenever I'll see you and part of me needs to prod myself by considering it and the other half needs to intrude on whatever it is you're doing to make it now. I surmise I'll decide to carry on."

Maybe this model from Lola Jean is somewhat of a significant piece, however would you be able to envision hearing this from your accomplice? Or on the other hand getting it by means of content? Will undoubtedly stimulate — and you'll be simply the one attempting to control from going to where your accomplice is. The fact of the matter is to entice, regardless of whether the situation being referred to won't really occur.

9. "I'm Thinking About Doing Many Things To You..."

"I'm pondering doing numerous things to you. None of them are acceptable. Well one of them, possibly — yet we shouldn't educate your mom concerning the others."

If you recently read that and said for all to hear, "WTF? For what reason are we bringing mother into this present," there's a clarification for it.

"A great deal of time we pay attention to dirty talk SO," Lola Jane says. "While it very well may be not kidding, don't be reluctant to stir up some outlandishness into it. The more you know the individual the more you can tailor that dirty talk to their specifics. When you don't realize somebody too dirty talk can be a brilliant spot to learn, yet track with alert instead of putting it all on the line right away." Remember: sex should be enjoyable.

10. "I Want You To Give Me So Much Pleasure I Lose The Concept Of Language, We Have To Use Our Bodies To Communicate."

Our bodies, how they react to contact, our outward appearances, our eyes — every last bit of it, often state undeniably beyond what words can, and that is not something to underestimate.

Saying, "I need you to give me so much joy I lose the idea of language, we need to utilize our bodies to convey," puts center around exactly how much our bodies express without words and it makes a degree of erotic nature, alongside the sexuality.

11. "The Next Time I Give You Pleasure, I Want You To Remember The Time Distinctly So..."

Extraordinary dirty talk waits. You can't shake it insane and in any event, when you set yourself back there you're probably going to get stirred. That is the reason tossing in an interest, while being somewhat controlling (in an attractive, consensual way) is an extraordinary strategy to utilize. As Lola Jean proposes, take a stab at saying, "whenever I give you delight, I need you to recall the time unmistakably so every time that assortment of numbers shows up on your telephone or watch you consider me."

There you have it — 11 sexually unbiased approaches to talk dirty. You can totally have a phenomenal, hot, scrumptious dirty talk meeting when you center around things that are driving you wild.

Utilize your words to turn him on.

Before I give you these dirty talking models, I first need to talk to you regarding why you ought to figure out how to talk dirty to your person just as how to talk dirty to your man viably with the goal that you stimulate him, manufacture sexual pressure, keep him pondering you and at last have an all the more satisfying sexual coexistence together.

For what reason would it be advisable for you to talk dirty to your man?

The most impressive thing it does is that it keeps your man contemplating you.

By utilizing dirty talk in increasingly inconspicuous, backhanded ways, your man will never be very certain what you mean and subsequently he will wind up continually pondering you and what you said. This is essential for keeping him pulled in.

Furthermore, talking dirty is amazingly hot and stirring to your man if you do it the correct way. As you can presumably figure this makes it extraordinary to utilize if you need to make sex more sweltering and more agreeable than expected.

In conclusion, what talking dirty to your person does is assemble sexual pressure. Sexual pressure is urgent if you need to keep your relationship from getting exhausting.

How would you make dirty talking some portion of your sexual relationship?

Before I go over what you should state, I need to tell you the best way to talk dirty adequately initially.

Numerous individuals imagine that it's what they state that has the effect, yet truly it's very you state it.

Consider this for a minute: if you go to your man with a silly smile and in a noisy voice you rapidly state, "I need you so awful," then it will sound somewhat odd.

However, if you gradually stroll toward your man, put your hand on his chest and look enticingly at him before utilizing a sultry, hot voice to murmur in his ear, "I need you soooo terrible at this moment" — then it will turn him on very quickly.

Notice the difference? One is very hot and a significant turn on for your man — the other is simply dreadful. It'll most likely have the contrary impact and turn him directly off.

Presently's simply an opportunity to dirty talk utilizing a portion of the accompanying recommendations.

What's more, FYI: these additionally work incredible via telephone or as sexting messages or even as immediate messages via web-based networking media like Facebook, Instagram and Snapchat.

Step by step instructions to talk dirty before sex:

1. "I need you at the present time."

2. "I get so turned on simply pondering the last time we had intercourse."

3. "I feel so frail and turned on simultaneously when I'm in your arms."

4. "I need to give you the best oral sex you've at any point had."

5. "I need you to gradually kiss me from my lips, down my neck, onto my bosoms and right down my body." (don't hesitate to rephrase this to something much dirtier if you're agreeable.)

6. "I simply need to be utilized by you today around evening time. Would i be able to be your own toy?"

7. "I can hardly wait until we're both alone so I can knock your socks off."

8. "I need to tie you up later and have my way with you."

9. "Feeling you over me and in control is the most sizzling thing ever!"

10. "I was pondering you the previous evening before I rested ..."

11. "I love the way you take a gander at me when we're as one, it's so hot!"

Step by step instructions to talk dirty during sex:

12. "Simply lie back and let me put everything in order."

13. "I love feeling you in my grasp!"

14. "Continuing onward, continue onward!"

15. "I love the amazing way you taste."

16. "Try not to stop, it feels so great!"

17. "You overwhelming me is such a turn on."

18. "I need you to assume responsibility for me."

19. "Quit talking and simply do me!"

20. "I never need you to stop, it feels so great."

21. "I need you to complete any place you like."

If you need to convey these lines viably, make sure to consider these things:

The tone of your voice. Here and there a profound and heartfelt tone is extraordinary for building sexual pressure and keeping him considering you, while different occasions a progressively energized, shifted tone works incredible for turning him on.

How quick you're talking. Talking gradually is quite often more impressive than talking immediately when talking dirty.

What you're doing with your body. If you tell your man, "I love your butt in those pants" however you are not in any case taking a gander at him and your non-verbal communication is totally cut off, then he'll realize that you don't generally mean what you are stating. In any case, if you keep in touch and are confronting him and contacting him – then it's going to considerably more powerful.

DIRTY TALK TO WOMEN

Have you at any point had dirty considerations about a young lady? Have you at any point needed to advise her precisely what you need to do to her until she's hot and sweat-soaked and prepared to hook your garments off?

All things considered, if I know most men, you've likely kept those considerations and words to yourself. You may have even retained them while you were connecting with a young lady for dread that she may get outraged and leave. However, try to keep your hat on, she's hanging tight for you to break out the dirty talk. So today I'm going to talk about how to dirty talk with ladies the correct way, and how to take your experience and hers to the following level.

I stared at her for a minute. Her eyes dashed down and away and started to dance about the room, however I brought her looking down as an away from of fascination. We were examining some everyday theme or another; the words were getting away into a cloudiness of vitality and a trade of vibes. Yet, the subtext trade couldn't have been more clear. Her students started to extend and her palms were getting sweat-soaked.

I snatched the rear of her head and pulled her toward me until my lips were inches from her ear. I realized she could feel my hot breath stinging the side of her face. I started kneading her scalp. I began to talk from my stomach, guaranteeing my voice was in any event an octave lower than typical. I seized a tight her other arm. I revealed to her that if we weren't in an open scene, I would pummel her in a bad position, pull her hair back and kiss her everything over her neck while I ripped her garments off. Also, before the night was finished, she realized that I was a long way from all talk. And keeping in mind that I was strolling the walk, I kept on dirtying talk with her until she really wanted to discharge the creature inside.

I've had a ton of involvement in dirty talk when either connecting with young ladies or sexting them. Maybe to an extreme, some could state. Yet, what I can let you know no ifs, ands or buts is that similarly that ladies love sex, ladies love dirty talk.
However, such a significant number of men are just hesitant to push the sexual envelope. They are worried about the possibility that that the lady will get awkward, or she will dismiss them, or they themselves will become awkward because they are wandering into a new area. In any case, in light of your faltering, I will share one of my preferred Mark Twain cites:

"Quite a while from now you will be increasingly disillusioned by the things that you didn't do than by the ones you did. So lose the anchor. Sail away from the sheltered harbor. Catch the exchange winds your sails. Investigate. Dream. Find."

If you've perused my pieces previously, you've heard me talk about my dread of "imagine a scenario where?" Cultivating this dread is the means by which I had the option to wreck approach tension. Getting dismissed, getting extinguished, missing the mark... everything can be extremely excruciating (until you in the end simply understand that you're realizing, that is), however nothing, and I amount to nothing, is more agonizing than lament. Realizing that as a man you could've accomplished something; you could've acted, yet you didn't do anything.

So sail away from your protected harbor and take a risk for once in your life. You have no clue how a lot of a young lady will regard you. What's more, you might be astounded at the outcome. Also, in particular: do it for yourself.

Fortunately for you, dirty talk is anything but difficult to learn, and an extraordinary spot to begin if you need to begin stretching the limits more.

Stage 1: BE A SEXY MAN

If you're attempting to dirty talk to a lady you've never laid down with, or hell, a lady you haven't had more than one discussion with, the possibility can be overwhelming. It very well may be frightening just to consider it. The truth of the matter is, when most men attempt to dirty talk to ladies, they appear to be:

Unpleasant

Clumsy

Uncaring

Excessively Aggressive

In any case, they fall off in these ways for reasons that you may not think. It's positively not because ladies don't care for dirty talk. They simply should be prepared for dirty talk.

If you put on a show of being excessively forceful: This implies you didn't appropriately set up a young lady to get sexual. This is particularly an issue for men of shading. You are seen as normally forceful, along these lines, simply dispatch into dirty talk and you'll be directly in accordance with that recognition, sending her into auto-dismissal. Much the same as really connecting with a young lady, you have to get her in the state of mind.

If you put on a show of being obtuse: This implies you shifted the state of mind to sexual when there was excessively "well disposed" of a vibe, or if you were profound plunging her and she was trusting in you. If a young lady is disclosing to you a genuine anecdote about how she lost her dearest youth little dog and you begin talking about how you need to get her bare, she'll simply feel like you're attempting to utilize her.

If you put on a show of being clumsy: This implies you set an awful point of reference with the young lady and your being sexual just left the blue. Or on the other hand, it implies that you haven't gathered up enough social speed and you're conveying uncomfortable vibes.

If you put on a show of being dreadful: This implies your non-verbal communication is clumsy, you haven't developed enough social confirmation in her eyes, you didn't give her conceivable deniability, and additionally your style/game is excessively powerless.

I don't normally prefer to praise silver projectiles, yet this is one of the occasions where I can say that these visual cues can be fixed by a certain something: improving and adjusting your provocative vibe.

If you're being seen as excessively forceful, your provocative vibe is excessively solid, and you have to dial it back with more energy and making her giggle/feel quiet so as to have her open herself up additional to your advances.

If you're experiencing being unbalanced or frightening, your attractive vibe is excessively frail. You have to take a shot at hitting young ladies with your provocativeness directly off the bat. You are putting on a show of being excessively "safe", and a young lady doesn't consider you to be a real darling alternative.

If you're experiencing being inhumane, your provocative vibe is confounded. You have to associate with the young lady on an enthusiastic level and cause her to feel like she's interfacing with you. And afterward you can alleviate the strain with a joke or some light prodding and begin to get sexual.

Stage 2: SUBTLE DIRTY TALK EARLY IN AN INTERACTION

Except if a young lady is simply started up and all set, you'll need to begin the dirty talk in a light and unpretentious manner. I was as of late bantering to and fro with a young lady and we were talking about work and snickering about entertaining proficient stories – nothing too naughty... until I tossed some unobtrusive sexuality in with the general mish-mash. I quit snickering and took a gander at her as though I needed to get her and maul kiss her at that moment. Then I got a slight grin all over.

Me: But that is only my normal everyday employment. You couldn't deal with what I do around evening time...

Her: [a sultry look in her eye] Oh definitely... and what might that be?

Me: I'm a janitor. Because I get dirty, I make things wet, and I deeply inspire individuals.

Furthermore, this line (and lines like these) did an astonishing thing for me. It was an explicitly charged line, so it made her go and in an increasingly sexual outlook. Be that as it may, after I said it, she really wanted to chuckle because it's only a clever line too. So it deals with two levels. Great inconspicuous sexuality imparts sexual subtext while keeping the outside layer of correspondence light and fun. Since she's giggling, she can't blame you for being unpleasant or excessively sexual, however since you did simply offer a sexual remark, she sees you more in the sweetheart casing. Sexual jokes, when utilized well, can be extremely useful assets for pushing a cooperation ahead.

Stage 3: ESCALATE TOUCH

I don't have to emphasize the significance of touch in the craft of enticement. So if you've been taking part in light sexual chitchat, this is an ideal opportunity to begin contacting her. You ought to be energetically contacting her while you exchange, and as you start to profound jump her and make the connection more substantive, you should begin utilizing the more delayed types of touch.

Stage 4: TURN UP THE HEAT

If you've built up an association with her, turn up the sexual warmth when she least anticipates it. Obviously, don't do it if she's simply revealed to you a genuinely charged story and is searching for your approval, yet do it when are talking about yearnings like travel, or are kidding around to alleviate the strain, or are simply examining a progressively unremarkable theme. For instance:

Her: And that was the insane story of my excursion to Bali!

You: Wow, that was a significant story! I'm going to call up National Geographic at the present time! Also, after all that, here we are in an arbitrary American jump bar. Isn't this the fantasy?

Her: Haha, I know right... this is the life!...

You: [grabbing her arm, and inclining in directly by her ear] Sarah, I need you to know, if we weren't right now, be kissing all over your neck at the present time, sliding my hands down your body and grasping a firm your hips. Also, I'd simply be beginning...

And afterward you pull back, stare at her for a second, and afterward keep talking regularly. And afterward propose setting off to a calmer spot or getting a nightcap or setting off to an after gathering, or whatever else goes to your head.

Fast note: if it's truly on, you don't need to return to ordinary discussion. You can simply disclose to her that you folks can get it going and leave at that moment. So this should be founded on your judgment.

Stage 5: THE AMAZING "NO SEX" LINE

I took in this line from a characteristic companion of mine. When I originally began utilizing it, its viability really bewildered me. Furthermore, what was considerably all the more stunning was that the more smoking the young lady was, the better the line became.

So it goes this way: while you're on the stroll back to your place or her place – or if it's less on, when you show up at your goal – you stop the young lady and get a genuine look all over. Then you look her dead in her eyes and summon up each ounce of sexuality that you have in your body.

We should make one thing straight...

Young ladies are sexual animals. Young ladies love sex. Young ladies consider sex, possibly more than you do. Young ladies, ladies, anything you desire to allude to the more pleasant sex as – they are not these unadulterated, chastised animals numerous in the media describe them.

I trust you definitely knew this, yet I needed to ensure we are in agreement. What's more, since you definitely know this, you ought to likewise realize that each young lady appreciates a touch of sexting every now and then. Particularly while she's ovulating. It's science.

Why You're Getting No Sexts

If you're perusing this article and thinking, "Gee, I wonder why I never get any sexts from young ladies?" then you've gone to the perfect spot. You're not getting any sexts because you're presumably doing one of a couple of things wrong.

Issue 1: Attraction Type

You may not be making enough fascination. Not the "goodness he's charming and perhaps I'll let him take me on a couple of dates" sort of fascination. I'm talking the "ohhhh crap! For what reason am I following this outsider into his condo" sort of sexual fascination.

If she's not explicitly into you, you most likely won't get any sexts, exposed pictures or dirty talking from her. You need to stir her so as to get dirty writings and photographs from a young lady. You can't simply pull in her. She needs to effectively consider your rooster somewhere inside her before she'll effectively draw in you in sexting. Furthermore, unmistakably, this is simpler after you've laid down with a young lady...

Issue 2: No Sex For You

You may not be getting sufficiently laid. It's constantly simpler to get stripped pictures and dirty writings from young ladies you've laid down with previously. You'll generally be playing a daunting task if you're attempting to get things warmed up before laying down with her. It's conceivable, however more difficult.

Issue 3: Tactless Thirsty Dudes

You don't have the foggiest idea Whether you need to how to talk dirty with her appropriately. You go from "0 to 100" way too rapidly. Rather than preheating the broiler, you're excessively ravenous (or parched). You toss it in on sear and afterward overlook the stove miss when you attempt to take it out. You have no tolerance or class.

Ladies love men of activity. They love men who follow what they need, however just if done in the best possible way. Continuously be a man of honor. You shouldn't ever appeared to be an audacious or inconsiderate social retard with no channel.

For instance, this is a terrible content to send to a young lady:

"Decent gathering you the previous evening, can hardly wait to f**k you sideways in the not so distant future"

There is no exchange. There is no being a tease. There is no sizzle. You appear to be parched. This young lady will lose the fascination she had for you if any whatsoever. She will think you think she is a prostitute and disregard you.

The most effective method to Talk Dirty To Girls Over Text (and ideally get some provocative shots)

Cautioning: The accompanying sexting models are very immediate, and we would prefer not to appear to be hostile. We accept that a man ought to endeavor to be however much gentlemanlike as could be expected and approach each lady with deference and profound respect. In any case, when it goes to the room, truly, isn't tied in with getting dirty?

Here you go:

Be Playful and Tactful, But Slow Down Until You Know Her

Presently we talked about being parched and utilizing class to get her heated up. You can toss all that out the window once you know a young lady. Everything is situational and once you know a young lady, you can pull off significantly more than with a young lady you don't know excessively well.

There is a scarcely discernible difference with gradually done idea. You would prefer not to appear to be an ordinary dweeb kind of fellow. You despite everything need to be the energizing sort of man she'll content. In this way, you need to be prudent, however energetic simultaneously truly.

For instance, with a young lady you had quite recently met the previous evening or a day or two ago, you could begin a discussion off explicitly with something like this:

"Great to meet you the previous evening... that provocative minimal bum of your is going through my head... completing no work today, you're a horrible impact on me!"

This model is fun loving and she'll appreciate the tease. You'll likewise certainly disclose to her you're a sexual man, not some pleasant, exhausting fellow – the sort of fellow she's presumably exhausted with.

Be that as it may, if you definitely know a young lady and engaged in sexual relations with her, you can truly begin things rapidly. This is a genuine case of a snappy discussion with a young lady you as of now have gotten physically involved with:

You: "Well it's Thursday evening, I'm off work and I'm so horny when I consider you... what would it be a good idea for me to do?"

Her: "Get some ice?"

You: "Senseless young lady, that is mischievous. You weren't honored with hips like that to no end... get the decent clothing, some red lipstick and get here at this point!"

This young lady is going to come over and go through an exquisite night ass exposed with you, as long as she doesn't have any too squeezing plans. You were reckless however diverting. You caused her to feel hot and sort of overwhelmed. You didn't put on a show of being a wet blanket. This is the means by which you dirty content.

butt

Start From the Beginning

Presently, the most ideal approach to begin a dirty messaging discussion is to begin from the earliest starting point. Be that as it may, you can't be an awkward wet blanket in doing as such. You can begin a discussion with a to some degree sexual vibe. This is because many folks abstain from being lively and sexual for the most part.

Start with the light wicked stuff and prop up from the absolute first content. Then consistently attempt and transform things into a sexual insinuation, regardless of whether it's a cheesy one. You don't need to talk about twisting her over a work area in the senior member's office to stimulate her.

For instance:

Her: "Hello you, how's your day going?"

You: "Gracious hello gingersnap... a touch of exhausting to be straightforward. Need some fervor today... "

Her:"Really? What sort of energy :)"

You: "Idk, perhaps an agreeable house cleaner who's does all that I ask... "

Keep the vibe fun and coy from here. You can keep sexting or you can push for a meetup.

You May Offend Her

You will in the long run annoy her. Or on the other hand one of your "hers" will get irritated. You will be dirty messaging and she will get resentful. This is fine. Simply don't be a colossal bitch and start saying 'sorry' in a penniless way. Mellow out play things cool. She may simply be trying you.

In any case, you have to give a little expression of remorse. One approach to do as such:

Her: "that was extremely discourteous"

You: "Ahhhh I didn't offend you really awful did I? Ugghhh fine, you get one punish and that is it... "

You acknowledge and recognize she is vexed, yet you don't bow down to her will. She despite everything regards you and you've kept up her fascination.

Jumping Deep – Dirty Texting For Experts

If you're a virgin and like to remain as such, you won't have any desire to keep understanding this. Notwithstanding, if you're prepared to take your sexting to the following level – read on.

Here are a couple of increasingly master dirty messaging tips:

Running The Questions Game Over Text

You should as of now be running "the inquiries game" on pretty much every first date. It's the most straightforward approach to plunge into more profound subjects and take a discussion sexual. Young ladies love that poop.

It's additionally a simple method to take a messaging discussion to a sexting discussion. Here's the specific system you should utilize:

You: "so wanna play a game"

Her: "Umm sure"

You: "Cool inquiries game. 3 inquiries each, yet you need to answer sincerely. No falsehoods or BS. You can't rehash the inquiry another person previously posed"

Her: "Hah alright however you ask first"

You: "I'm a man of honor. Women consistently start things out"

Presently a dominant part of the time she'll battle you on this. That is fine. You can contend somewhat to and fro. She may ask first or she may "make" you.

If she asks first, answer every one of her inquiries genuinely and give her criticism if they are exhausting. If they are sexual, you're set. If she gives you exhausting ones (and is a held young lady) and you replied, you then mirror her inquiries while including a touch of edge. When she answers, give criticism and afterward cycle two. She may start to sexualize or she may not. When you find a workable pace second round, you do.

If she "makes" you ask first, you can turn it on her rapidly:

You: "Well I was going to get along, yet since you're in effect so obstinate... "

Try not to hang tight for her reaction:

You: "1. What number of men have placed their rocket into your she pocket?"

You: "2. Do you like being commanded in bed?

You: "3. What's the one sexual thing you've for the longest time been itching to attempt yet never had the nerve to do?"

These are the cash questions. You need to find a workable pace the game. They are what is important. So – regardless of if she goes first, you go first, the vibe isn't sexual...

You need to find a workable pace. She might be shy, however she'll reply. Flippantly get down on her about anything that doesn't sound genuine. Spitball a piece on her answers, then state

You: "Your turn"

She'll ask you in any event a couple of sexual inquiries, generally every one of the three. Answer truly, yet offer admonition to her if anything is "as well" odd or insane before advising her (model: you've had 200 sexual accomplices).

Run one progressively adjust and pose two sexual inquiries dependent on her answers (model: What turns you on the most? How would you generally come?). Toss in an inquiry dependent on her youth too. You need it to be sexual, yet light. Something like:

You: Did you ever find a good pace greatest pound in middle school?

She'll reply. After two rounds, you ought to have enough things to content about. Let the inquiries game part of the sexting vanish.

In the wake of making her warmth up, you can request nudes if you think all is good and well.

Messaging Her To Orgasm

You can utilize this after the inquiries game or in a different circumstance. If you have a young lady who is sexual from the hop, a young lady you've laid down with previously or a young lady with whom you've appropriately raised the convo, you can calmly offer to walk her through a climax.

When she's somewhat worked up, from some kind of sexting you can say:

You: If you ask pleasantly, I may simply let you have a climax.

Her: Umm not certain what you're talking about, however sure

You: Say please and evacuate your jeans.

Her: Ok and please

You: Good young lady. Presently envision I'm there...

You: over you. I've nailed you down against the bed. I'm going to take you while you squirm and groan in delight. You feel a shiver between your legs as my hand contacts you. I get a clench hand brimming with your hair and pull you close before kissing you profoundly. My fingers go through your hair as we kiss.

You: Then I get you and through your hands behind your back and curve you over. SMACK. You feel my hand give your rear end a firm smack. You whence as you groan. You feel a sting, however a nice sentiment as well. I take my belt and limit your options together.

Her: gracious wow

You: you need more?

Her: yessss

You: I push your face into the pad and pull my hand back to punish you once more... this time hard. You howl in torment, however the cushion suppresses your groans. I instruct you to quiet down and take it like a decent young lady.

You: I flip you over and push you on you knees. I stand up and look at you without flinching before making you suck my hard chicken as I stand. You take my hard cockerel in my mouth as I powerfully get your hair. I begin to push a greater amount of my chicken in your mouth as you choke.

Her: ahhh this is acceptable

You get the thought folks. You simply keep messaging her dirty until she says she's regarding to come. Then reveal to her you didn't let her yet. After a couple of more sexts, you end one with:

You: "Cum. Presently."

The key is to warm her up before finding a good pace, reveal to her you'll make her come. When she's warm, be extremely unequivocal and prevailing in your writings. Then don't let her come until after the peak of your sexual story. That is when you utilize the last content.

Don't hesitate to request naked photographs, particularly if she came.

Requesting Photos The Right Way

A few young ladies will simply send you photographs unexpectedly. A few young ladies will never send photographs. A few young ladies will just send photographs to folks they've engaged in sexual relations with. A few young ladies will spam photographs to everyone.

If you've warmed her up through content, you are in a situation to request photographs. When she's warmed, you can pull off pretty much anything as long as you don't send "nudes" or something weak like that.

In any case, possibly you've engaged in sexual relations with a young lady, yet haven't been sexting a lot. You need to get bare photographs of her, however might not have the opportunity to put resources into a lot of sexting. In addition, she's not the sort to simply send nudes for reasons unknown or unexpectedly.

Whenever you shag her, offer it to her great multiple times and be harsh with her. Ensure you finish a piece sweat-soaked and exhausted. As you finish, you'll need to turn over and tap your chest. She'll move her head on your chest and you'll cuddle a piece.

Give her a light kiss on the temple and gradually recapture your breath. Then commendation whatever piece of her body you need photographs of, yet state it in an exasperated way:

You: "God, you have a decent screwing ass."

Or then again...

You: "Fuck, your tits are great."

You then slap her rear end and get her tit. Delicately. You would prefer not to intrude on the postcoital cuddles.

What's more, recall – the commendation must be veritable.

She won't overlook it, particularly if you screwed her right.

Presently, you may discover she sends you a photograph of her rear end as well as tits inside seven days of this event (once more, contingent upon how well you screwed her). If she doesn't, you have set yourself up to request a bare.

Start a discussion. It very well may be ordinary, yet ensure things are somewhat perky. Then bring it up:

You: "For reasons unknown that bum of simply yours won't leave my brain. It's screwing tormenting me. I can't rest. I can't eat ;)"

Her: "Haha that is not my shortcoming. You're the wicked kid ;)"

You: Ahh well I can't deny that, however I do know a pic or three of that bum may help with the entire eating and resting"

She may not send them immediately, yet she will in the end. Because you asked pleasantly.

One key thing to recollect: if you've found a workable pace in the discussion with a young lady, you can and often should, stack these dirty messaging tips. For instance, you can begin by running the inquiries game to sexualize the discussion. Then idea to walk her through a climax. When she's done, you could demand a couple of bare photographs as a much obliged.

DIRTY TALK TO MAN

Today you will figure out how to talk dirty to your man to make him rock-hard for you.

Regardless of whether you are right now single, in a long haul relationship, or even wedded, you should know a few deceives on the most proficient method to pull in a person, and keep the sentiment and the science between both of you alive.

Realizing how to talk provocative and dirty to your man, sharpening those abilities to flawlessness, and later really applying them in your affection life, can be both animating and energizing.

Attractive dirty lines as an incredible asset

Attractive dirty lines, when utilized accurately, can assist you with drawing a person like a moth to a fire. Nonetheless, if you don't have a clue what you're doing, the entire thing can reverse discharge and flop hopelessly.

There is no requirement for me to dive into insights concerning your sexuality and attractive dirty talk. This serves just to engage you so you can relinquish your limitations and completely make the most of your sexuality on your standing.

What's a superior method to communicate and investigate the points of confinement of your sexuality than to figure out how to talk dirty to your sweetheart.

Well you need not stress as right now step I will tell you precisely the best way to talk dirty to your man.

Vital prescience about people before you gain proficiency with the craft of dirty talking

Before you begin finding out about how to talk explicitly to a man, there is something you have to think about the two people.

Sonnet by Victor Hugo - "Man and Woman"

"... Man is the flying bird.

She is the songbird that sings.

Flying is a predominant space. Sing is to vanquish the spirit.

The man is a Temple.

The lady is the Tabernacle.

Before the sanctuary we find ourselves, we stoop before the Tabernacle.

In short: the man is set where the land closes.

The lady where paradise starts."

Acing True Sexual Pleasure With The Help Of Dirty Talking

As per Dr. Ava Cadell, proficient speaker, essayist, and sex advisor in Los Angeles, Calif., couples take part in dirty talk to "increase their excitement and offer dreams that they might not have any desire to transform into the real world, however talking about them can be shockingly better."

Sex in mix with the ideal and energetic sweetheart leads you headed for encountering sexual delight and unadulterated rapture consistently.

Following that way will take you to finding and understanding the genuine significance behind sexual joy and love. It will clarify your brain and contemplations.

Also, dirty talk is perhaps the most ideal approaches to upgrade your sexual delight and satisfy your sexual dreams

Today you'll find and completely ace the specialty of lovemaking and sexual delight with the assistance of dirty talk.

I need you to make each stride right now talk manage gradually and consistently to get a handle on the center idea of talking dirty to a man.

When you ace this center idea you'll be presented to an a lot further and increasingly significant degree of sexual and mental fulfillment in your relationship.

The purposes behind learning and applying these dirty lines

Remember that by perusing and utilizing the dirty talk lines won't just set you up for sexual joy yet in addition for the ceaseless and future love and warmth from your man for quite a while.

Rehearsing these systems and adhering to the guidelines on talking dirty to him, you will immediately turn into the ace of the ideal love making which will lead you to the spots you have never been and take your relationship to another level.

Consolidating extreme and energetic love with fantastically convincing and prevailing sexual joy will make your relationship a lot more grounded and stable.

Utilizing the attractive expressions from this article will turn your sweetheart on and cause him to hunger for you more than ever.

Get to know his sexual inclinations

An examination led by the internet dating office, Saucy Dates, has uncovered that both, types of people, love commotions and words during sex.

So for this dirty talk to do something amazing for your sweetheart, you should initially get to know his sexual inclinations as opposed to talking dirty to him right away.

Answer the inquiries.

Just by noting a few straightforward, yet powerful inquiries, you will have the option to comprehend and find out about what he different preferences during a sex. Those inquiries are the accompanying ones:

Does he like to be predominant when it comes to sex?

Does he act forcefully, harshly and like your proprietor?

Does he lean toward being agreeable?

Does he utilize antagonistic language and irate or debilitating reactions?

Which body some portion of yours stands out for him the most?

It is safe to say that he is firmly pulled in by incredible entertainers and fundamental characters?

Do famous people he's pulled in to have the equivalent or comparable highlights?

An unobtrusive and straightforward young lady nearby, a wild lady, with solid sexual nearness or absolutely honest?

The most effective method to Combine His Sexual Fantasies With Dirty Talk To Blow His Mind

Finding out pretty much all the sexual dreams he's shared, which are the most widely recognized topics he prefers, and what are his most shrouded wants?

Is it to be revered like a lord, associated with an undertaking, or to rule a solid and influential lady?

Has he at any point had the accompanying sexual dream?

A case of the most well-known sexual dream:

The silk scarf tied around my wrists was cutting into my skin. In spite of the fact that the blindfold was closing out all of light, I despite everything had my eyes shut. An unexpected sharp spot of my left areola made me howl in delightful torment.

"Shhhh, Baby You aren't permitted to make clamor. Do it again and I will beat you!" he said. I pondered opposing him. . . just to savor the smack of his hand against my rear end. However, before I could open my mouth and state something I felt the tickle of a plume running up my internal thigh and afterward our lips squeezed together in an enthusiastic kiss.

Unexpectedly, he stops and pulls away. I am feeling lost and befuddled not realizing where he'd gone. In any case, this was all piece of the game. Halting and beginning. Hard and delicate. Torment and delight.

My faculties were on alarmed and honed not realizing what's in store straightaway. He could tell I was restless so he consoled me. "I love watching you so turned on and needing me.

Gesture your head if you need me at the present time." I needed to be cool however I shook my head enthusiastically and began shouting yes. I was unable to see it, yet I swear I could feel his grin broadening. "Presently spread your legs as wide as could be expected under the circumstances so I can embed my penis. Hold them like that until I reveal to you that you can move" All I could do was to comply.

I was totally uncovered. My arms and legs were attached to the bed. I was totally bare with my legs spread as much as I could.

Defenseless. Terrified. . . be that as it may, I consented at any rate. Furthermore, that was exciting and energizing.

In this way, enough with the sneak peaks!

Women, if you are prepared, how about we get familiar with the expressions that drive men wild and talk dirty.

1. Coquettish (and marginally dirty expressions) known as consideration grabbers

It is ideal to begin simple and utilize basic and coy expressions on your man. Simply dunk your toes in the water to perceive how sending a dirty instant message works out for both of you and whether it will get you need you need.

Have a go at sending something like this:

1. Stop. . .

- diverting me
- turning me on, I can't focus
- filling my psyche with wicked considerations
- pondering me. Return to work

2. Mmmm...

- I am thinking some extremely yummy things about you at the present time
- I continue thinking about your astonishing kisses
- you are terribly adorable, you realize that?

3. Are you. . .

- reddening? You ought to be, founded on what I'm thinking.
- rested up? I intend to deplete you on Saturday.
- turned on as am I? Stunning.

4. Damn...

- contemplations of you make them grin today
- I am so turned on by you
- I can hardly wait to be sleeping with you

5. Know what?

- I can hardly wait to feel your kisses.
- You are one hot beau.
- I just escaped the shower. Appreciate that visual.

6. Can I simply let you know. . .

• your arms are damn hot

• you have me turned on

• how great you looked an evening or two ago?

7. Disclose to me something. . .

• do we look great together for sure?

• for what reason would you say you are so damn enticing?

• what amount would you say you are anticipating next time?

Content him this dirty lines to consume his brain until whenever he sees you (make them consider you)

1. What might you do. . .

• if you were here the present moment?

• if I was there with you?

• if we were separated from everyone else at the present time?

2. I can't quit pondering. . .

• how my body reacts to your touch.

• the things I need to do to you.

• the things I need you to do to me.

• the entirety of the spots I could kiss you.

3. Envision this. . .

• me running my fingers through your hair as we kiss and you getting so rock hard down there.

• me snacking your neck and gradually working my mouth down your body

• you contacting my delicate skin, investigating my neck. . . shoulders. . . back. . .

4. I can hardly wait to. . .

- feel your body by mine, skin to skin. . .
- jump on you when I see you!
- have you in my bed, alone, and continuous. . .
- make you my attractive love slave
- run my hands over every last trace of you and make you cum.

His answers may inspire a scope of feelings and sexual strain. After perusing your messages, he will be stirred and prepared for you immediately.

Be that as it may, if things gain out of power at the very beginning, don't stress, you don't need to partake if you think it is unreasonably best in class for you.

You can generally utilize some cooling sex expressions, for example,

- Whoa there! We should spare some for some other time.

Be that as it may, if you would like to flavor it up a piece and take part in cutting edge dirty provocative talk, then utilize any line of the accompanying:

- Oh you are so shrewd.
- Slow down sir, a lot of time for those exercises.
- I have you truly turned on huh? Shrewd me.

And afterward separation yourself from him saying you need to come back to work, or meet your companions or simply make sense of another motivation to walk out on him. Anything that will stop the discussion.

He won't realize what hit him and conceivably respond peculiarly and unexpectedly. If, some way or another, his response is real and sweet, then take a stab at keeping things closer to the PG-level only for the time being.

2. Sext-starter – The best dirty talking lines to use on your sweetheart

The most ideal approach to begin the discussion is with a lively sex talk message that asks for his reaction. Something that will make his creative mind go out of control:

- If you were here. . .
- I wish. . .
- Guess what I'm doing. . .

• Stop. . .

• Know what?

• You have me soooo. . .

The ellipsis utilized after the expression won't just keep him fascinated and inquisitive about what follows straightaway yet additionally let him know there is something else entirely to the idea.

He will assuredly be confounded by your dirty and unusual content, however over the long haul, he will know he's in for a treat.

What he can anticipate from you when he gets such dirty provocative message is a sizzling sex shock.

The sext-starter will make his creative mind go crazy.

From that point forward, by talking explicitly to your man, you can control the discussion any bearing you wish.

You can attempt to hop immediately by sending him a sexting "fast in and out" or start gradually and progressively advance into his heart and bother him into talking explicitly with you.

Here is the means by which you can dirty provocative talk to your man

3. Sexting Quickie – Hot and Steamy Messages

When you have assembled some involvement with talking dirty to your man, you can utilize something nastier and at last unusual, so the accompanying lines are perfect for you:

1. If you were here. . .

• I'd stroke your hard chicken and imploring you to screw me.

• I'd be face down, ass up on the bed so you could top me off so profound.

• you'd make the most of my tight, wet kitty feline. purrrrrr. Mmm.. .

• my pussy is so prepared for you, infant

• I need to fold my mouth over your rooster at this moment

2. You have me sooo. . .

• horny at this moment. I need you to screw me terrible.

• turned on and wet, omg I need to feel you inside me, screwing me hard.

4. Fun loving and Innocent Sexy Texts

If you aren't happy with the nastier stuff, then you can generally return to fun, energetic and honest approaches to content your beau.

1. If you were here. . .

• I would meet you at the entryway absolutely exposed.

• I wouldn't have the option to keep my hands off of you.

• you'd see exactly how wicked I'm in the state of mind to be. Extremely underhanded.

2. I wish. . .

• I could feel the heaviness of your body over mine at this moment

• you could feel precisely how turned on I am at this moment

• you and what's in your jeans were before me this second.

3. Mmmmm.. .

• do you have any thought how turned on I am by you?

• the considerations I'm having at the present time. Is it true that you are reddening? You ought to be.... .

• I am aching for your touch right currently child

And afterward, when you have made a casual air, you can take swift, decisive action by sending him nastier messages as:

If you were here. . .

• I would take you in my mouth, licking and sucking until you lose control.

• you could twist me over the rear of the lounge chair and take me. . . rigid. . . the subsequent you stroll in the entryway.

• you could pour nectar all down my stripped body and lick it allllll off. . . inch by inch.

2. Stop. . .

• making me so horny. I can't complete any work considering what I need you to do with my body.

• filling my head with delightfully dirty thoughts (then proceed to depict).

3. You have me sooo. . .

• turned on. I need you within me, topping me off, making me groan sooo terrible at the present time.

• wet at the present time.

5. Clear and direct messages for dirty provocative talking

Being clear and direct will get you to places you need. Sending these profoundly enticing dirty provocative writings will hit the dead center.

Be direct and let him know precisely what you need him to do to you OR what you need to do to him.

Take a stab at sending something along the lines of:

• I can hardly wait for you to... in my... .

• I can hardly wait for you to gradually disrobe me taking a gander at me with your attractive room eyes.

• I can hardly wait for you to snack my areolas. Licking, sucking, a touch of gnawing. Do you realize how hot that gets me?

• I can hardly wait for you to give me your hard chicken in my eager pussy.

• Tonight I'm heading off to... your... until you...

• Tonight I'm going to stroke you with my hot wet tongue until you go over the edge with delight.

• Tonight I'm going to suck your chicken until you cum.

• Tonight I'm going to ride you until you cum so hard infant.

• I need you to... my... until I'm...

• I need you to lick my clit until I'm squirming and groaning and peaking.

• I need you to screw me from behind until I'm making such a lot of clamor I wake the neighbors.

- I need you to go down on me until all aspects of my body is shaking with delight.

- First, I'm going to... Then I need you to...

- First, I'm going to torment you with a moderate, provocative strip bother.

- Then, when you can't control yourself for one increasingly second, I need you to have your way with me.

- First, I will jump on my knees, unfasten your jeans, and bring you profound into my mouth. Then I need you to look as I do something amazing until you detonate.

- First, I will slather whipped cream all over my tits. Then I need you to take as much time as necessary as you lick everything off.

These are only a couple of essential recipes that make it simple for you to begin.

Also, as should be obvious from the models, some of the time you need to change them somewhat so they bode well for the specific bearing you are giving.

As you become agreeable, by all methods release your inventiveness and work out your own unequivocally specific writings!

Second Book: TANTRIC SEX

WHY DO WE HAVE SEX

Your accomplice may concoct twelve reasons to state "Not today around evening time, dear, I have a _____," yet what number of reasons can you two name for needing to engage in sexual relations?

One? Two? Twenty? What about 200? Some undergrads have refered to upwards of 237 different explanations behind having intercourse.

From delight to reproduction, weakness to curiosity - the present purposes behind taking a move in the roughage appear to change as much as the terms for the deed itself. A 2010 Sexuality and Culture survey of sex inspiration considers expresses that individuals are offering "unmistakably more explanations behind deciding to take part in sexual movement than in previous occasions." And we're doing it all the more often as well. It's a conspicuous difference from recorded presumptions, which refered to just three sexual intention: To make babies, to feel better, or because you're infatuated.

Today, sexual practices appear to have taken on a wide range of mental, social, social, even strict implications. However, some sexologists state, at the most essential level, there is just one genuine explanation individuals look for sex.

Wired for Sex

"We are customized to do as such," sex specialist Richard A. Carroll, partner Northwestern University psychiatry and social sciences educator says. "Inquiring as to why individuals have intercourse is similar to inquiring as to why we eat. Our minds are intended to persuade us toward that conduct."

The possibility that people are hard-wired for sex mirrors a developmental point of view, as indicated by University of Hawaii brain research teacher Elaine Hatfield. "Transformative scholars bring up that a longing for sexual relations is 'wired in' so as to advance species endurance," she says. "Social scholars will in general spotlight on the social and individual reasons individuals have (or keep away from) sex. Societies differ uniquely in what are viewed as 'fitting' explanations behind having or maintaining a strategic distance from sex."

What's Your Motive?

For what reason do you look for sex? Inspirations for the most part fall into four fundamental classes, as indicated by therapists at UT-Austin who asked in excess of 1,500 undergrad understudies about their sexual mentalities and encounters:

Physical reasons: Pleasure, stress help, work out, sexual interest, or appreciation for an individual

Objective based reasons: To cause a child, to improve societal position (for instance, to get well known), or look for vengeance

Enthusiastic reasons: Love, duty, or appreciation

Weakness reasons: To help confidence, shield an accomplice from looking for sex somewhere else, or feeling a feeling of obligation or weight (for instance, an accomplice demands engaging in sexual relations)

The Difference Between the Sexes

As a rule, men look for sex because they like how it feels. Ladies, in spite of the fact that they may likewise get joy from the demonstration, are commonly increasingly inspired by the relationship improvement that sex offers. Scientists portray these differences as body-focused versus individual focused sex.

Body-focused sex is when you engage in sexual relations because you like the manner in which it causes your body to feel. You aren't worried about the feelings of your accomplice.

Individual focused sex is when you engage in sexual relations to associate with the other individual. You care about the feelings in question and the relationship.

"Men often begin being body focused," says University of Hartford assistant brain research teacher Janell Carroll. "Yet, that changes later on. As men arrive at their 40s, 50s, and 60s, their relationship turns out to be increasingly significant."

Richard Carroll has been guiding couples with sexual issues for over two decades. "Ladies really become progressively like men after some time in that often, at an opportune time, sex is tied in with starting, creating, strengthening, and looking after connections, however in a long haul relationship they can really concentrate on delight."

Notwithstanding these general perceptions, look into additionally proposes that there has been a major assembly in sexual perspectives among people as of late. In 1985, Janell Carroll and associates found that most school matured guys had easygoing sex for physical reasons without enthusiastic connections. She rehashed a considerable lot of a similar report inquiries to another crowd in 2006.

"Rather than people being at far edges of the sexual range, they are presently meeting up," she says. "More ladies may be having intercourse for physical reasons, yet a lot more men were bound to state they had intercourse for enthusiastic reasons."

20 Reasons People Have Sex

Worried? Have intercourse. Stress decrease is one of the main reasons Americans, especially men, state they engage in sexual relations, Richard Caroll says. The survey, distributed online in Sexuality and Culture, shows other most every now and again refered to explanations behind having intercourse include:

Boosting state of mind and assuaging wretchedness

Obligation

Improvement of intensity

Improvement of self-idea

Encountering the intensity of one's accomplice

Feeling cherished by your accomplice

Encouraging desire

Improving notoriety or economic wellbeing

Bringing in cash

Making babies

Requirement for friendship

Nurturance

Accomplice curiosity

Friend weight or weight from accomplice

Joy

Diminishing sex drive

Vengeance

Sexual interest

Demonstrating adoration to your accomplice

Otherworldly greatness

Why Study Sex?

Understanding why individuals look for sex isn't constantly a straightforward assignment. Most investigations have included school students, an "example of accommodation" for college specialists however one that is often exceptionally restricting. Youngsters and ladies ordinarily haven't been in exceptionally serious relationships and are finding their sexuality. Their responses to "for what reason do you engage in sexual relations" are often significantly attached to the picture of themselves and their social connections, says Richard Carroll. This can change after some time.

Be that as it may, such information can improve a couple's sex life.

"Understanding these differences in inspirations is significant. It encourages us comprehend what's happening in the sexual relationship and treat sexual clutters. All the time, you discover the wellspring of the issue can be followed to the specific inspiration," Richard Carroll says.

If you need assistance, you can locate a qualified sex specialist in your general vicinity through associations, for example, the American Association of Sexuality Educators, Counselors and Therapist (AASECT) or The Society for Sex Therapy and Research.

BOOSTS YOUR LIBIDO

Moxie, or sex drive, normally changes between people. Having a low sex drive isn't really an issue, however if an individual wishes to help their moxie, they can attempt a scope of powerful characteristic techniques.

Uneasiness, relationship difficulties, wellbeing concerns, and age would all be able to influence drive. While a low moxie isn't normally hazardous, it can influence an individual's connections and confidence.

Right now, look the absolute most ideal ways that guys and females can build their drive utilizing characteristic strategies.

Common approaches to support drive

The two guys and females can help their charisma utilizing the accompanying techniques:

1. Oversee tension

Ordinary exercise and open correspondence can help forestall tension influencing drive.

Having significant levels of uneasiness is a typical obstruction to sexual working and charisma for the two guys and females. This might be uneasiness because of life stress or specific sex-related nervousness.

Individuals with a serious work routine, caring duties, or other life stresses may feel exhausted and, accordingly, have a low sexual want.

Tension and stress can likewise make it progressively difficult for somebody to get or keep up an erection, which can put an individual off engaging in sexual relations. A 2017 audit of erectile brokenness in youngsters has recommended that downturn and uneasiness can bring about a diminished moxie and expanded sexual brokenness.

There are numerous things that individuals can do to deal with their nervousness and lift their emotional wellness, including:

rehearsing great rest cleanliness

setting aside a few minutes for a most loved leisure activity

practicing routinely

eating a nutritious eating regimen

attempting to improve connections

conversing with a specialist

2. Improve relationship quality

Numerous individuals experience a respite in sexual want and recurrence at specific focuses in a relationship. This may happen in the wake of being with somebody for quite a while, or if an individual sees that things are not working out in a good way in their close connections.

Concentrating on improving the relationship can expand each accomplice's sex drive. This may include:

arranging date evenings

doing exercises together outside of the room

rehearsing open correspondence

saving time for quality time with one another

3. Concentrate on foreplay

Having better sexual encounters may build an individual's longing for sex, in this way boosting their drive. Much of the time, individuals can upgrade their sexual encounters by investing more energy in contacting, kissing, utilizing sex toys, and performing oral sex. A few people call these activities outercourse.

For ladies, foreplay might be particularly significant. As indicated by nearly 2017 research, just around 18 percent of ladies climax from intercourse alone, while 33.6 percent of ladies report that incitement of the clitoris is essential for them to climax.

4. Get great quality rest

Getting great rest can improve an individual's general state of mind and energy levels, and some exploration likewise interfaces rest quality to moxie.

A little scope 2015 investigation in ladies recommended that getting more rest the prior night expanded their sexual want the following day. Ladies who detailed longer normal rest times announced preferable genital excitement over those with shorter rest times.

5. Eat a nutritious eating regimen

Following a nutritious eating regimen can profit individuals' sex drive by advancing great dissemination and heart wellbeing, and by expelling specific nourishments that can diminish charisma.

Metabolic disorder and cardiovascular ailment can influence physical sexual working. Likewise, polycystic ovarian disorder can influence hormone levels, which may likewise disturb drive.

Eating an eating regimen wealthy in vegetables, low in sugar, and high in lean proteins can help forestall scatters that influence moxie.

6. Attempt natural cures

Examination into the advantage of maca powder for moxie is progressing.

There is little examination into how compelling home grown cures are at improving sexual capacity in guys and females, however a few people may discover them advantageous.

A 2015 survey study expresses that there is constrained however rising information that the accompanying home grown cures may improve sexual capacity:

- maca
- tribulus
- gingko
- ginseng

Individuals ought to be careful about utilizing home grown drugs without their primary care physician's endorsement. Some home grown meds can communicate with existing prescriptions, and the Unites States Food and Drug Administration (FDA) don't manage them. Thus, their quality, immaculateness, and wellbeing stays indistinct.

7. Get normal exercise

Getting normal exercise can help charisma from multiple points of view. A 2015 investigation of men experiencing androgen hardship treatment, which brings down testosterone levels, found that ordinary exercise helped men adapt to issues, for example, self-perception concerns, low drive, and relationship changes.

A 2010 survey of ladies with diabetes refers to inquire about indicating that activity may help lower diabetes-related side effects in ladies. The investigation accentuates that doing activities of the pelvic floor might be helpful in ladies without diabetes.

8. Keep up an empowering weight

A few researchers interface overweight and corpulence to low sex drive, alongside different variables identified with diminished ripeness. This is related with hormonal elements, for example, low testosterone focuses.

A few people who are overweight may likewise encounter mental impacts, for example, lower body certainty.

Keeping up a solid body weight can improve an individual's sex drive, both truly and mentally. Eating a stimulating eating routine and getting standard exercise can help accomplish this, just as lift an individual's general energy levels.

9. Attempt sex treatment

Sexual want is unpredictable, with both mental and physical segments. In any event, when an individual has a physical condition that influences moxie, for example, diabetes, improving the enthusiastic and mental reaction to sex can improve charisma and sexual working.

Treatment is a viable methodology for expanding low moxie. Singular directing can assist address with negativing sees about sex, confidence, and optional reasons for low drive, for example, gloom and tension. Relationship directing can assist some with peopling work through components influencing their sexual want.

Close by talking treatments, care treatment may likewise help. One 2014 investigation found that only four meetings of care based subjective social treatment in a gathering setting improved sexual want, sexual excitement, and sexual fulfillment for ladies.

To locate a reasonable specialist in your general vicinity, search the AASECT registry.

10. Stop smoking

Smoking cigarettes can negatively affect an individual's cardiovascular framework. Great heart wellbeing is significant for acceptable sexual working.

Individuals who smoke cigarettes may find that their energy levels and sex drive increment after they quit.

The common methodology

Hoping to flavor up your sex life? There are an assortment of things you can do in your regular day to day existence that can help support your charisma and upgrade your sex life.

1. Take a stab at eating certain natural products

Little proof backings the adequacy of specific nourishments, yet there's no damage in testing.

Figs, bananas, and avocados, for instance, are viewed as moxie boosting nourishments, known as aphrodisiacs.

Yet, these nourishments likewise give significant nutrients and minerals that can expand blood stream to the privates and advance a solid sex life.

2. Have a go at eating chocolate

Since forever, chocolate has been an image of want. Because of its heavenly taste, but since of its capacity to improve sexual delight.

As indicated by one investigation, chocolate advances the arrival of phenylethylamine and serotonin into your body. This can create some love potion and temperament lifting impacts.

As per another investigation, the impacts of chocolate on sexuality are presumably more mental than organic.

3. Take your day by day herbs

Next time you choose to plunk down for a sentimental supper, include a little basil or garlic to your dish. The smell of basil invigorates the faculties. Garlic contains significant levels of allicin, and builds blood stream.

These impacts may assist men with erectile brokenness.

Ginkgo biloba, a concentrate got from the leaf of the Chinese ginkgo tree, is another herb found to treat upper instigated sexual brokenness.

4. Take a tip from Africa

Yohimbine, an alkaloid found in the bark of the West African evergreen, has been referred to function as a characteristic Viagra.

A few investigations propose that Yohimbine bark can assist you with keeping up an erection. It will likewise improve the nature of an erection. Nonetheless, specialists state there is no characteristic proportionate to coordinate Viagra.

5. Lift your fearlessness

The manner in which you feel about your body influences the manner in which you feel about sex. An unfortunate eating regimen and absence of activity may make you have a poor mental self-portrait. These things can dishearten you from having and getting a charge out of sex.

You can help your confidence and your sex drive by shifting the concentration from your imperfections to your properties. You can likewise concentrate on the joy experienced during sex.

Boosting charisma in guys

Testosterone substitution treatment can improve charisma.

Charisma in men is often identified with testosterone levels, which will normally decay as men age. Testosterone substitution treatment can support a few men.

In men with testosterone insufficiency, or hypogonadism, testosterone substitution treatment can bring about improved drive, diminished gloom, and improved erectile capacity, as indicated by one 2017 audit.

There is little proof to propose that specific nourishments or enhancements increment an individual's testosterone levels and sexual capacity. Some examination proposes that zinc, nutrient D, and omega-3 unsaturated fats might be significant dietary segments for testosterone.

6. Stick to one glass of wine

Two glasses of wine may be one too much. Drinking one glass of wine can comfort you and increment your enthusiasm for getting personal. Be that as it may, a lot of liquor can destroy your capacity to perform by influencing erectile capacity. An excessive amount of liquor can likewise restrain your capacity to climax.

7. Set aside some effort to think and calm pressure

Regardless of how sound you are, being worried is going to influence your sex drive. Ladies are especially vulnerable with the impacts pressure can have on one's sex life.

Men, then again, some of the time use sex to ease pressure. Furthermore, once in a while differences in the way to deal with sex may cause struggle.

To soothe pressure, take an interest in sports exercises, practice jujitsu, or take a yoga class.

8. Get a lot of rest

Those with a tumultuous lifestyle don't generally have the opportunity to get the perfect measure of rest. Being occupied additionally makes it difficult to set aside a few minutes for sex.

Individuals who offset work with thinking about maturing guardians or small kids are often left depleted, which can prompt a decreased sex drive.

Lift your energy and sex drive by taking snoozes when you can and eating a solid eating regimen high in protein and low in starches.

9. Hold your relationship under wraps

After you've had a contention with your accomplice, odds are you're not in the state of mind to have intercourse. For ladies, detecting passionate closeness is essential to sexual closeness. That implies uncertain clashes can influence your sexual relationship.

Correspondence is basic for building trust. It's imperative to keep feelings of disdain from working up.

Counsel a specialist

Regardless of whether you're adopting a characteristic strategy to boosting your sex drive, it despite everything may be a smart thought to converse with your primary care physician. They can assist you with identifying basic issues.

Your primary care physician may propose a few methodologies for improving sexual wellbeing.

These may incorporate speaking with your accomplice, settling on solid lifestyle decisions, and treating fundamental ailments. Knowing the foundation of the issue influencing your sex life will make it simpler to discover an answer.

Experimentation

There are a wide range of approaches that may upgrade your sex drive normally. Nonetheless, it's imperative to recollect that each couple is different. It might take a little experimentation to discover what works best for you.

If you do choose to go to physician recommended drugs, recollect that longing is at the center of sex. It's essential to recollect that a little blue pill may not be the appropriate response if intense subject matters are influencing your drive.

DEFINITION OF TANTRIC SEX

What is Tantric sex?

Tantric sex is an old Hindu practice that has been going for more than 5,000 years, and signifies 'the weaving and development of vitality'.

It's a moderate type of sex that is said to build closeness and make a brain body association that can prompt amazing climaxes.

Tantric sex – or Tantra as it's often known – should be possible by anybody keen on rebooting their sex life and finding new profundity to their affection making.

If that sounds confounding, consider it thusly – if fast in and out sex is what might be compared to a takeaway, tantric sex is a Michelin-featured feast, gradually and affectionately arranged and even more heavenly gratitude to the pause.

For what reason would it be a good idea for me to check out Tantric sex?

Tantric specialists accept that if you broaden the time and exertion you put into sex, you will arrive at a higher and progressively extraordinary type of delight.

What's more, it clearly works, because celebs, for example, Tom Hanks and Sting have said how extraordinary it is. Truth be told, Sting's wife Trudie Styler once broadly flaunted that her significant other could have intercourse for over 5 hours one after another!

Tantric sex is beneficial for you if...

– You're searching for something new to do in bed

– You need to turn out to be significantly increasingly close with your accomplice

– You need to attempt to reconnect with your significant other or beau

The most effective method to perform Tantric sex

The uplifting news is Tantric sex isn't 'objective arranged', which implies you don't need to take a stab at realizing what to do.

Try to take your psyche off your climax and rather center around making foreplay pleasant and compensating until you're prepared to take it to its regular end.

This is more difficult than one might expect obviously, so to postpone climax Tantric sex specialists utilize an assortment of strategies including reflective systems, breath control and back rub.

Tantric sex: What to do

If you need to give it a go, attempt the accompanying:

– Start by turning down the lights and closing out the remainder of the world.

– Loosen your body: Tantra is tied in with moving vitality through the body, so master Louise Van Der Velde proposes 'shaking your appendages enthusiastically to invigorate and unblock your framework before you start'.

– Stay off the bed: This will trigger the rest button in your cerebrum, which, as indicated by Louise 'signifies you'll be agreeing to a fast in and out cavort rather than profound association and adoring sex, which is at last what Tantra is about.'

– Get settled: Try resting with your accomplice on the floor and gradually begin to contact one another, taking as much time as is needed to lackadaisical advance around their body.

– Experiment: Try an assortment of contacts – firm back rub, light padded contacts, and delicate stroking. The point here is to elevate his faculties in a moderate and serious manner with the goal that you're building him to a pinnacle yet not taking him as far as possible and the other way around. Acted in the correct manner this can drag out sex and your pleasure for a considerable length of time.

– Think about breathing: If you discover your brain begins to meander, re-center around your relaxing. Breathe in as your accomplice breathes out and the other way around – it can help improve the association among you and keep your psyche on what's going on.

– Don't surrender: If you don't last past 10 minutes, attempt once more. Tantric sex sets aside some effort to find a workable pace because we're completely used to sex in a western manner – this implies we anticipate that sex should have an undeniable beginning, center and end.

With training you can relinquish this thought and appreciate sex without considering the end well as have the option to control your body so you can postpone peak and increment the quality of your climaxes.

Tantric sex works out

As Tantric sex is about closeness between two accomplices, the accompanying activities can assist you with getting a hang of Tantra:

1. Attempt the heart breath to tune into one another. Remain inverse each other and investigate each other's eyes setting your left hand on your accomplice's heart. He should then place his hand over your left one and you should attempt to coordinate each other's relaxing for at any rate two minutes.

2. Sit vis-à-vis (this works better if you sit in his lap). Wrap your arms as firmly around each other and press your body against one another. This sort of skin contact advances more prominent sentiments of closeness.

3. Guarantee you move and inhale gradually during sex (it can assist with maintaining a strategic distance from any position that you know makes you climax effectively) and move in the direction of a slow develop of joy. The more gradually you can permit your sentiments and sensations to develop, the more exceptional your inevitable climax will be.

PLEASURE AREA

When it comes to erogenous zones, it isn't about the touches, stubs, and cuts. Here are some far-fetched delight focuses that are often neglected.

Scalp

The scalp is brimming with nerve endings, and even the smallest brush of the hair can send shivers through your body.

To amp up the joy, run your fingernails delicately over the scalp, giving uncommon consideration to the space behind the ears and simply over the neck.

Remember about the hair. Delicate pulling can send influxes of joy through the body.

Ears

With delicate skin outwardly and several tangible receptors within, the ears top the rundown of erogenous zones for some individuals.

For some sexy aural activity that is certain to if it's not too much trouble attempt delicately kissing, licking, or snacking your accomplice's ear cartilage.

You can likewise exploit those tangible receptors by murmuring or daintily blowing into their ear for all the more tingly feels.

Navel and lower stomach

Being hazardously near the private parts makes this zone particularly stirring.

Utilize your tongue, fingertips, or even a plume to follow hovers around the navel and bother your way down and all around the stomach.

This is an incredible spot for some temperature play, so utilize an ice block if your accomplice is into it.

Playing solo? Touch the territory to get yourself in the disposition.

Little of the back (sacrum)

It could have something to do with the way that the nerves right now the spine are associated with the pelvis or the defenselessness factor of being contacted from behind that makes this territory so delicate.

Whatever it is, the smallest touch here can bring out delight. Stimulate the zone with a quill or your lips and tongue.

Feeling bold? Attempt an ice shape, a vibrator, or pinwheel for some tactile play.

Internal arms and armpits

Figure armpits can't be sexy? Two words: "Filthy Dancing."

You realize that scene where Johnny runs the rear of his hand down Baby's arm, touching her armpit?

She snickers from the outset, however once she moves beyond the stimulate reaction, it's absolutely hot.

A light touch is all you have to turn the tickle to absolutely titillating. Run your fingertips, your tongue, or even a quill gradually along the internal arm to the armpit.

Inward wrist

Home of the beat point and not used to getting a great deal of activity, the inward wrist is profoundly touchy.

Stroke the skin with your fingertips while taking a gander at your accomplice intriguingly from over the table, or anyplace else so far as that is concerned, when attempting to set the mind-set.

As of now in the throes of energy? Take a stab at entwining your fingers with theirs and brush the skin on their internal wrists with your lips and tip of your tongue.

Palm of hands and fingertips

The fingertips are the piece of the body most sensitive to contact, and your palms aren't a long ways behind.

Spot your hand under theirs with your palm looking up, and stimulate their palm with your forefinger.

If you need to up the closeness, keep in touch while you do it.

You can kick it up a billion indents by taking every one of their fingers into your mouth, individually, and sucking softly.

Behind the knee

This is another often dismissed territory that is fantastically delicate to any sort of touch. It's even sensitive for a few.

Give the zone some extraordinary consideration during a back rub, or utilize your mouth and tongue there before stirring your way up or down the leg.

A portion of these might be really self-evident, however others may very well astonishment you.

Areola and areolas

Areola incitement illuminates a similar region in the cerebrum as the private parts.

Start with a light touch, and anything goes here. Lips, tongue, a quill, or a little vibrator are only a couple of thoughts.

Follow around the areola before moving onto the areola and sucking, licking, and in any event, flicking. Blow or utilize an ice solid shape for some sexy cool.

If your accomplice likes it unpleasant, touch the areola with your teeth. Even harsher? Attempt areola cinches.

Mouth and lips

Kissing is a craftsmanship, and we propose utilizing every last trace of their lips and mouth as your canvas.

Follow the state of their lips with your tongue before moving to a moderate, wet kiss, or tenderly suck or snack on their base lip.

Fun truth: There are scientifically demonstrated medical advantages to kissing, so pucker up.

Neck

When it goes to the neck, even the smallest touch can make your whole body shiver.

Fold your arms over your accomplice, and run your fingernails along the rear of their neck, moving to the territory behind the ears before advancing around the front.

Proceed onward to delicately kissing the sides and front of the neck before working your way to the lips or traveling south where it's considerably more smoking.

Internal thighs

The internal thighs are so touchy and very near a definitive erogenous zone that even only a brush can set your flanks burning.

Run your fingertips down the front of the thighs, gradually moving your direction internal while you kiss their lips, neck, and chest.

When you're prepared to find a good pace individual, cover the region in delicate, wet kisses and licks.

Base of feet and toes

Weight focuses in the base of the feet can build blood stream and improve sentiments of excitement when controlled perfectly.

Test with different weights when rubbing the feet, beginning light and working your path more profound until you find what works.

If you're both into it, switch back and forth among kneading and licking the foot. Proceed onward to tenderly sucking each toe, individually.

The ones you're certainly mindful of

These may appear to be really self-evident, however the vaginal and penile locales contain various different erogenous zones inside them. How about we plunge right in, will we?

Vaginal locale

Pubic hill

The mons pubis, the beefy hill simply over the clitoris, is wealthy in nerve endings that are associated with the private parts. Rubbing the territory in a here and there movement can by implication animate the labia and clitoris.

If your accomplice is responsive to additional, proceed onward to kissing the region, then utilize the tip of your tongue to lick your way down. If you're playing with yourself, back rub or vibe to up your excitement.

Clitoris

This little delight bud contains more than 8,000 nerve endings and is secured by a hood. Delicately take it between your file and center finger and slide it gradually in a here and there movement.

Need more? Utilize your fingers or a clitoral vibrator and rub your stub utilizing light weight. Examination with course and beat to discover what feels best.

For some great tongue activity, start moderate and speed up and pressure.

A-spot

The lower some portion of the vaginal opening is brimming with sensually charged nerve endings and home to the front fornix (A-spot).

Use fingers, a dildo, or penis to infiltrate the vagina, and spotlight pressure on the front divider while sliding in and out.

G-spot

The G-spot is a territory equipped for causing what's known as female discharge. Fingers or a bended G-spot vibrator are your most solid option for arriving at it.

With a decent measure of lube, turn your vibrator or finger upward toward the navel and move it in a "come here" movement.

Find what feels better and keep at it, permitting the sensation to assemble.

Cervix

An individual should be completely excited to appreciate cervical incitement, so foreplay is an unquestionable requirement.

Any profound infiltration sex position can do it. Doggy style is a decent one that can be performed utilizing a tie on or customary dildo, as well. When you discover a profundity and movement that feels better, continue onward.

Cervical climaxes are like what's known as a full body climax in tantric sex, so you're in for a treat if you can arrive.

Penile district

Glans

The glans penis is what's known as the head. Because of 4,000 nerve endings, it's the most touchy piece of the penis.

Bother it by scouring your wet lips tenderly over the plump head before utilizing the tip of your tongue around the edge. Next, bring the glans into your mouth, whirling your tongue around it.

An all-around lubed hand can likewise do something amazing.

Frenulum

This is the versatile bit of skin on the underside of the penis, where the pole meets the head. It's exceptionally delicate and the essential trigger of climaxes in individuals with penises.

Hands or mouth — it's all acceptable here.

To get helpful with it, slide your lubed hand here and there the pole, letting your thumb brush the F-spot. During a penis massage, ensure your tongue gives additional consideration to this problem area.

Prepuce

The prepuce is loaded up with nerve endings that really upgrade delight for those with uncircumcised penises. This flimsy layer of skin gives the chance to blend it up for different sensations during a hand occupation or penis massage.

You can let it coast over the penis and organs with each stroke or tenderly withdraw it to concentrate on the stripped F-spot and head. Be delicate and use lube.

SPIRITUAL PHASE OF SEXUAL ENERGY

To manifest your full sexual vitality you need to give up. Its absolutely impossible around it. You should totally occupy your body and be at the time. If not currently, when? Keeping down, focusing on execution, or letting your brain drift is the finish of energy. Try not to go there. I'll tell you the best way to escape your head and into your happiness.

What is genuine sexual vitality? I characterize it as gladly asserting your suggestive self and carefully directing sexual vitality. You never use it to hurt, control, make victories, or get dependent on the self-image excursion of exotic delight to the detriment of others. This is terrible karma. Nor do you permit others to damage or lack of respect you. Sexual vitality isn't exactly what your identity is sleeping, however that is a part of it. You likewise make electric linkages to your body, to soul, to a darling, to the universe. For me, it's a turn-on when sexual force is mixed with profound force.

An excessive number of us right now, world come up short on the rich experience of having a basic association with somebody. Sexual vitality can offer us this, a fulfillment you can never get from your acumen alone. As you open to both sex and soul, regardless of whether you're single or part of a couple, you'll be a vessel for sexual stream, getting a charge out of delight without uncertainties or restraints.

We'll talk about numerous enjoyment approaches for giving up that you can incorporate into your lifestyle. Try not to stress if you can't succeed constantly. Be content with all of progress. Here are some broad tips to remember to improve your sexual vitality. The more you can rehearse them, for short or longer periods, the more sexually alive you'll be.

Essential Strategies of Surrender

+ Surrender your schedule, setting aside a few minutes for erotic nature and lovemaking.

+ Surrender your overactive, basic "monkey mind" that executes energy and prevents you from being available in your body.

+ Surrender to delight as totally as would be prudent.

+ Let yourself dissolve into the delight of climax and become one with your accomplice.

Sexual vitality is something to love and deliberately develop. You can't simply leave it to risk. When I find a good pace morning, the principal thing I do is contemplate. I need to interface with myself, to each ounce of otherworldly vitality, heart vitality, and suggestive vitality in me. I do this before any of life's requests meddle. Ruminating right now me and leaves me alone completely present. Being in contact with my sexual self is a piece of being available, alongside being logical or being thoughtful or tuning in to the heavenly attendants sing. Sexual force isn't compartmentalized away from all of you. It is progressively present when you're entirety. In this way, to start the day, I offer a debt of gratitude is in order for each part of me, then continue into the extraordinary obscure of the hours ahead.

we'll investigate questions, for example, How would you be able to touch off sexuality and have progressively serious climaxes? What makes a decent sweetheart? What are the regular enemies of energy? Do you dread closeness or do you counterfeit climaxes? What is the difference between sound holding and excessively connecting to an accomplice? Is it true that you are a sex fanatic? Do you lose your middle around sexual vitality or fixate on darlings? Do you oppose delight?

I'll tell you the best way to give up if you experience difficulty giving up or fear losing yourself in somebody. Giving up becomes simpler when you confide in your accomplice. Then you'll feel more secure about letting down your gatekeeper and feeling joy without obstruction or dread. There are no restrictions to where delight can accept you as your sexual vitality permits you to associate with yourself and an accomplice profoundly.

Guarantee Your Sexual Energy

Sexual vitality has different angles. In the most fundamental sense, it's about proliferation and endurance. Nature has cunningly wired us to be remunerated with suggestive energy when we propagate the species. The euphoria of climax is the catnip that persuades us to replicate. Our decision of an accomplice is firmly affected by our organic programming. Research has indicated that the two people are pulled in to sound, ripe mates with great qualities. What physical signs show this? Science has identified a few: a mate's thick hair, smell by means of hormones called pheromones, voice tone, facial balance, a man's strong physical make-up, and a lady's hourglass figure with a midsection to-hip proportion of 7:10 (which Marilyn Monroe had). Strikingly, when ladies ovulate, they produce copulins, a fragrance that pulls in men making their testosterone rise. Our drive to reproduce bests most other human senses. The intensity of this basic cognizance orders regard and wonder.

Another part of understanding sexual vitality between two individuals is enthusiastic closeness, an instinctual want to cling to a sweetheart, to feel comfort, to be known. This has the effect between unadulterated physical sex and lovemaking. Enthusiastic closeness originates from warmth, from sharing sentiments, from being powerless. Via mindful, you fortify each other's engaging quality and cause each other to feel uncommon. As companions and sweethearts, you are in a general sense there for one another which makes trust. You consider each to be as genuine individuals, the great and the terrible, not some admired form. When struggle, outrage, or hurt sentiments emerge you're focused on working through them. Carry your feelings of dread and uncertainties to an accomplice in an undefended manner. When you share all pieces of yourself, even your mysteries, you can genuinely give up. Tantric sexuality instructor David Deida

says to offer your feelings "from the most profound spot of adoration's desires that you can possess." With passionate closeness, you're fit for investigating enthusiasm on each level. Without it, there's a breaking point to where you and your accomplice can go. In the short run it might appear as though less difficulty to maintain a strategic distance from strife yet your suggestive life follows through on a cost. You can't tap your full sexual force if parts of you shut down. When you constantly shroud your sentiments, you sit around idly and open doors for closeness. If you remain open, in any case, your passionate love will upgrade your arousing love.

It's conceivable to have sexual closeness without passionate closeness yet you will utilize just a small amount of your sexual vitality. In any case, as I've seen with specific patients, a considerable lot of whom had alcoholic or damaging guardians, they may not feel meriting love. One man let me know, "I truly needed love however I agreed to sex." Sometimes, however, sex is all individuals look for or can endure. Regardless of whether they're mindful of it or not, they connect passionate closeness with mystic torment or being choked out which executes their sensual excitement once they truly find a good pace. When they draw near to an accomplice they begin feeling overpowered and turn off. "Ladies are continually requesting beyond what I can give," one male responsibility phobe let me know. Giving up to cherish feels terrifying to him. Such individuals have never discovered that correspondence can securely carry you closer to somebody than even a sexual vitality trade. In this way, so as not to work up the mammoth, they should keep a sheltered good ways from genuine closeness which easygoing uncertain sex permits.

Take my patient Roxie who originated from a harsh home and grew up a hard-bubbled Hollywood road punk. Solid and decided, she made another life for herself and assembled a fruitful sexy unmentionables organization. At thirty-five, Roxie was a connecting with blend of road savvy, hip, and entertaining. She had her own image of sexual vitality which she appeared quiet with. During our first meeting she shared, "My beau is an extraordinary darling. We keep it fun and light. Getting overwhelming remains things." With this disposition, it's reasonable that Roxie's connections never kept going over a half year. In spite of the fact that Roxie wasn't stressed over being single, she'd come to me because of an exceptional dejection in spite of numerous sentiments.

During treatment Roxie started to get a handle on that when feelings get genuine, her sexual vitality closes down. Previously, she'd essentially justify, "I'm simply not pulled in to that person any longer." Intimacy was Roxie's specific vulnerable side (everyone has one). She didn't understand that because of her harsh childhood, closeness didn't have a sense of security. My job isn't to pass judgment on anybody or to push patients to change before they're prepared. If individuals are content with their lives, God favor them. In any case, Roxie wasn't. All things considered, we needed to step delicately. Quite a while in the past, I figured out how to work with where a patient is at, then go from that point. Roxie wasn't yet prepared to impart her feelings to a darling. It was excessively undermining.

Along these lines, first, to facilitate her depression, I urged her to investigate different types of closeness, for example, kinships and getting a little dog—creatures are ace educators of unequivocal love. Then she could work her way toward closeness with a darling. Roxie found that loving her shih tzu came more effectively than offering authentic feelings to people. In any case, step by step she began trusting in companions and letting down her "nothing pesters me" intense young lady veneer to hazard being powerless. I additionally helped her perceive how she'd protected herself as a kid with the goal that she wouldn't feel hurt by her scattered split dependent guardians. Presently, after a year, Roxie is trying out her new passionate aptitudes with a mindful, marginally tense school English teacher—her direct inverse, which loans the ideal equalization. She relaxes him up; he focuses her. They've been as one eight months and the sexual vitality between those two individuals is acceptable. I am hopeful. Roxie has begun to recuperate the injuries that prevented her from giving up to an accomplice.

If you need to find all the elements of your sexual vitality, a relationship without enthusiastic closeness and trust won't be sufficient for you. Closeness includes give up, a longing to relinquish dread. You and your accomplice will intrepidly investigate the internal space of feelings together. Sharing feelings—not unnecessarily, however as they normally come up—is a piece of the stream. Lovemaking is about liberality and offering delight to one another. It's not just about you and your pleasure, significant as that seems to be.

Be that as it may, even past the natural and enthusiastic features of closeness, sexual vitality is bigger than simply your wants. It likewise includes tapping a higher force. There's an otherworldly nature that impels the entirety of our body's base drives. Nothing about being human is at any point simply physical notwithstanding what our brains or private parts let us know. Sexuality and soul are personally related. When you give up sexually, you enter an open natural state, allowing the power of creation to course through you, like how specialists are moved. Therefore, you may actually make another newborn child life or you might be rebirthed yourself.

During sex, conventional limits fall away and your cognizance is changed. You experience the happiness of the extraordinary. You can naturally detect things about one another. When you give up, you are a channel. I'll tell you the best way to work on welcoming soul wherein thus triggers the body's biochemical delight reaction. With age, otherworldliness and unobtrusive vitality keep sexual force alive. Enthusiasm of the body is aroused by the energy of paradise. Realizing this is the start of knowing ecstasy.

What makes a decent darling? There's an electric science between couples that is extraordinary to them. Smell, voice, contact, and kissing style all figure in. Specialized abilities and great cleanliness are significant also. Yet, past these, here are a few attributes to search for.

10 Qualities of a Good Lover

1. You're a willing student.

2. You're energetic and enthusiastic.

3. You cause your accomplice to feel sexy.

4. You're sure, not reluctant to be powerless.

5. You're brave and ready to explore.

6. You convey your necessities and tune in to your accomplice.

7. You set aside a few minutes and don't surge.

8. You appreciate giving delight as much as you appreciate accepting it.

9. You're strong, not critical.

10. You're completely present at the time with great eye to eye connection and can give up.

What prevents us from being acceptable sweethearts? As often as possible it's time limitations, conceit, restraints, and absence of system. Our psyches won't shut off which shields us from being at the time. Further, a considerable lot of us oppose giving up to how sexy we truly are. Why? We haven't figured out how to consider ourselves to be sexy. We've been mentally conditioned by the "thin perfect."

Additionally, sex is often seen more as a presentation accomplishment than as a sacred sexual vitality trade. Growing up, the vast majority of us haven't been given the correct sort of instruction about what genuine sexiness is. If just we'd been encouraged that sexuality is a solid, characteristic piece of us that we should encapsulate in a careful, cherishing way—not something "grimy" or something to be embarrassed about. At an early stage we discover that the words "vagina" and "penis" humiliate individuals. Aside from between sweethearts, they are seldom part of our jargon. We are a culture that grasps disgrace, just there is not something to be embarrassed about!

At sixteen, when I was going to have intercourse with my beau of two years just because, a life-modifying transitional experience, I got some information about sex. Looking stricken, as though I'd recently detached her heart, she set some hard boundaries: "Judith, it's extremely soon. How about we talk about this when that is no joke." End of story. I surmise Mother trusted that by declining to examine it she'd prevent me. She was unable to have been all the more off-base. I felt a balance of remorseful, frantic, and defiant, hell bent on doing what I'd arranged. I would not like to hurt Mother, yet from my perspective, this wasn't about her—it was about me. I realized she was worried for my government assistance however not tending to my sexuality wasn't useful.

I wish guardians and authority figures would at long last handle that when you tell young people that sex is illegal, it coaxes even more. It then gets perilous, hazardous, all the more profoundly charged. Many refined guardians today get this. They genuinely talk about the upsides and downsides of high school sex without disgracing their kids or cutting them off. Otherworldliness should be a piece of that conversation. Two spirits sharing suggestive enthusiasm through a sexual vitality trade is a method for commending soul as well. Realizing that a mindful (not rebuffing) higher force is included brings worship, uprightness, and obligation to having intercourse for the two adolescents and grown-ups. It hoists the experience. Soul is upbeat that we love one another. It has numerous sides, including sexiness. If just we were trained that sexuality supplements otherworldliness by connecting us with a more noteworthy power of affection, that they're not at war with one another. How different our perspectives would be!

Similarly as child chicks engrave on their moms, we engrave on our folks. You were blessed if your folks demonstrated a sound sexuality and instructed you to be pleased with your body. My patients who've been raised like this are increasingly OK with themselves and with giving up to their sexuality. Deplorably, for all of us, such confidence about our bodies is hard-earned. In any case, utilizing the accompanying systems, you can relinquish negative programming. Considering yourself to be a sensual being and grasping your own charm are the compensations of enlivening sexual vitality.

In some cases, however, we oppose our own sexiness or having intercourse at all because it reflects our uncertainties. Normal ones incorporate "Is my body appealing? Is my accomplice making a decision about me? Am I a decent sweetheart? Will I frustrate my accomplice? Will I be dismissed? Choked?" When these or different feelings of trepidation dominate, even intuitively, you may oppose your sexual vitality. Obstruction can manifest as genuine reasons, for example, "I'm not in the state of mind," "I'm excessively worn out or run down," "I'm engrossed with work," "It's an excess of exertion," "The children will hear," or "I have a cerebral pain." Still, if these reasons become constant and your suggestive life is enduring, it's fundamental to look at your protection from sex.

There are useful advances you can take to defeat opposition. You need to need to be sexy and keep enthusiasm alive in a relationship. When you're worn out or furious, or if correspondence with your accomplice separates, enthusiasm rapidly vanishes. Refusal and lack of concern are the adversaries of energy. So remain alarm to the accompanying obstacles to a decent sexual vitality trade. Then you can address the circumstance.

Regular Killers of Passion

1. Depletion

2. Not imparting your requirements

3. Losing interest

4. Hurrying

5. Absence of imagination, weariness

6. Stifled indignation and threats

Sexual responsiveness is a delicate indicator. Closeness requires mindfulness and an eagerness to evacuate obstructions. Making a move can assist you with accomplishing a cherishing, sensual relationship. Consistently, train yourself to be progressively careful about getting rest and finding a steady speed. It's not sexy to surge around and be continually worried. Particularly when you're occupied, it's critical to make sure to inhale—a brisk method to reconnect with your body. Despite the fact that family, work, and different requests can interfere with setting aside a few minutes for sexual vitality, being committed to self-care can assist you with organizing it in your relationship.

To fix self-questions, you should be arrangement situated. For example, if you wonder, "Is my system right?" genuinely talk with your accomplice about how you can address each other's issues. If you're exhausted with similar positions, energetically conceptualize together about energizing approaches to explore. Likewise, with deference, continue talking about the indignation or hurt you may feel toward one another so your feelings of disdain don't numb energy. For progressively complex issues, for example, dread of closeness, connect with a specialist or a companion for knowledge. While investigating your feelings of trepidation, be caring to yourself. Such sweetness permits you to patch wounds and recover your sexual force.

Give up to The Ecstasy of Orgasms: Explore Sacred Play

Climax is the crown gem of give up. You tap into the early stage stream of life just as discharge strain. The more given up you are, the more happy the climax.

Sex and climaxes are an inherent piece of being human. For me, these are the extraordinary compensations of having a body! The World Health Organization appraises that in any event a hundred million demonstrations of intercourse occur every day around the world. (All things considered, American couples engage in sexual relations two times each week. The normal male climax keeps going ten seconds and a female climax is twenty seconds or more.

holy sexuality-hymn isadora

I could scarcely accept the national surveys uncovering that about 50 percent of ladies report having climaxes inconsistently or not in any way during intercourse. Additionally, various examinations have discovered that ladies counterfeit climaxes up to a fraction of an opportunity to ensure their accomplices' emotions. These measurements feature a glaring hesitance a significant number of us must be straightforward with our accomplices about our sexual vitality trades. We'll talk about how give up, an essential information on life systems, and a little skill can improve correspondence and upgrade climaxes for both sexes.

What is a climax? How could this supernatural occurrence ever be only a certain something? It includes physical, enthusiastic, otherworldly, and fiery gives up. On a physical level, when you're sexually stirred, your climax releases strain, bringing about musical pelvic withdrawals and delight, even elation. In men, climax regularly happens from animating the penis; in ladies, from invigorating the clitoris or the hallowed G-spot in the vagina. These pieces of our body are brilliantly touchy because of a high thickness of nerve filaments. Stroking them actuates joy focuses in the mind. Your body shifts gears. You inhale more earnestly. Your pulse increments. Blood hurries to your private parts, making them swell. At peak men, and a few ladies, discharge. Endorphins, the common "feel-better" hormones, flood your framework. You experience floods of joy, stress vanishes, and a warm gleam penetrates your body.

The Erotic Ecstasy of Foreplay

Foreplay is an open door for couples to stir and support one another however ladies appear to need it more. It's a method to fabricate sexual vitality as opposed to just discharging it. The normal man can include a climax inside a couple of moments or less. Ladies may require as long as twenty minutes of foreplay. Preferably, obviously, neither one of the partners hears a clock ticking. Numerous couples I treat are in heaven letting sexual vitality strain mount before intercourse with no feeling of time. Foreplay lets them feel close, investigate, play, draw out the euphoric aches of excitement.

I compare foreplay to tuning an instrument. You have to feel it instinctively, and the sexual vitality between two individuals, find the perfect touch, the correct kiss, and sense how you and your accomplice's bodies react. I grinned when I as of late observed a man in a bistro whose T-shirt read, "I will work for sex." True, it might require more exertion for a lady to climax however that is what being a decent sweetheart methods: realizing how to satisfy somebody without surging, getting joy from one another's pleasure. Then foreplay never just feels like work. What's more, here's a basic anatomic truth: nature didn't put the clitoris (in contrast to the penis) in the immediate line of entrance. During foreplay it should be physically or orally animated except if the edge of your bodies happens to be perfect, which is more uncertain. Most ladies can't have a climax with intercourse alone. Couples must know this so they can commonly delight one another.

If a man needs to win a lady's heart, the time and the delicacy he places into foreplay assist her with giving up during sex. She can't be surged. A typical issue I've seen with couples in my training is that if a man is spent, he might need to have sex absent a lot of foreplay, then simply nod off since discharging makes him tired. I'm not saying a lady can't appreciate a fast in and out now and again however when all is said in done this training doesn't bolster an enthusiastic relationship. I urge couples to straightforwardly talk about the problem of adjusting the entirety of life's requests, to consent to make an effort not to slip by into the trench of quick ones. Then they can design sensual intermissions to relaxed appreciate each other during a sexual vitality trade and the delights their bodies bring to the table.

To upgrade foreplay, attempt the following activity to stir your faculties and let go to delight.

Exercise: Surrender to Your Senses

Put aside continuous time to try energetically. Start to unwind by breathing profound and slow. We routinely inhale shallowly to temper sexual and different sentiments. I need you to detect, not think, to be completely in your body.

Stir contact. Take a new blossom or a plume and tenderly stroke each other's bodies. (For me, it's a rose in full blossom with petals going to fall.) Start with the face, neck, chest, bosoms, and the heart zone, step by step advancing down to the privates. Rehash fragile, roundabout movements over these regions. They react to a light touch. It'll feel stunning and energizing. Give up. Revel in the sensations.

Stir taste. Select a couple of nourishments, herbs, or flavors that have punch. Organize them on a plate. My top choices are papaya, peppermint, and nectar. I have a patient, a specialist with a relentless psyche, who livens up her sexual vitality by enjoying a succulent bit of watermelon. To increase your feeling of taste, I recommend wearing an eye veil or a free blindfold, maybe produced using a silk scarf. Then, with eyes secured, have your accomplice offer you every choice individually. The tongue is a sexy supernatural occurrence of sensations. Let the joy of taste spread all through your body. Permit it to stir each pore.

Stir smell. Presently, investigate smell. It is a cozy and significant piece of sexual vitality, one that can turn you off or on. Let a blindfold emphasize your investigation of this sense. One patient, a full-time mother, gets an erotic lift from a couple of whiffs of lavender or gardenia oil during the day, and she keeps them helpful in her work area and vehicle. Test out different aromas. Perceive how your body reacts to the fragrances of different herbs, oils, or aromas. Use them as a sexy boost.

Play with development and shaking. Investigation with moving your bodies together to manufacture sexual vitality. Shaking your bodies while holding each other can be incredibly exotic. Likewise, when you first observe each other in the wake of being separated, a long, quiet grasp or embrace joined with shaking is stirring. Moving or unconstrained freestyle developments are beautiful as well.

Check out nature. Attract on nature's enthusiasm to uplift your sexual vitality. Tempests, fog, rainbows, wind in the forested areas—appreciate whatever states of mind of nature energize you. Let them stir your body. Know about hues, surfaces, sounds. Assimilate them all. For example, I'll whirl on my overhang to the erotic tone of a far off foghorn, getting one with it and the sea close by. Arousing quality can be transmitted from nature to you, an unconstrained assimilation if you permit it to occur.

This activity intensifies your own sexual vitality and the suggestive connection among you and your accomplice. Investigating each other is never only a one-time occasion. Continue finding the subtleties of one another's affectability and style. Analysis with what gives you both goose pimples, shivers, or floods of warmth. Notice how your body feels, every last bit of it. This lets you experience more delight and closeness.

There Is No Such Thing as Casual Sex

From an instinctive point of view, your climax is never simply your own during lovemaking. Sexual vitality gets transmitted to your accomplice, influencing their prosperity. Your vitality fields cover, passing on both bliss and depression (in any event, during brief hookups). From that viewpoint, there is nothing of the sort as easygoing sex. Actually, my touchy patient Pete favors not to have intercourse with his wife if she's furious about work. Sensibly enough! He's glad to hear her out vent when she gets back home however if she's despite everything sticking to the resentment when they engage in sexual relations, it gets transmitted even without talking it. This doesn't feel great to Pete and channels him. Such vitality move between couples often occurs, however most don't know about it. I need you to be. During climax standard limits obscure. You're helpless. Your heart opens. In the best of circumstances, climax is a trade of vitality that favors the two accomplices. The French call it le petit mort or "the little demise," a complete give up that slings you and your darling into the blissful arms of the awesome.

Tantra is a powerful Hindu framework that shows the craft of suggestive love by joining sex and soul. Westerners often consider sex to be direct, the objective being climax, yet tantra sees sexual love as a ceremony and a vitality trade between two individuals. As per tantra, climax isn't just a physical discharge. Utilizing specific positions, you move sexual vitality upward from the private parts to support and purify your entire being.

It's enjoyable to know about sexual vitality during lovemaking. Vitality is radiated through the eyes: the exotic way you see somebody can stir the person in question. Eye to eye connection is an approach to remain associated with your accomplice. Additionally during climax, when vitality rises, you may free awkward feelings. I've had various (generally male) patients state, "My accomplice once in a while cries when we have intercourse. Have I accomplished something incorrectly?" I clarify, "In the two people, crying and snickering are enthusiastic discharges, indications of enthusiasm, nothing that necessities fixing." Tantric instructor Barbara Carrellas calls unconstrained chuckling during sex "giggleasms." Check out these responses with your accomplice. Except if the person says differently, there's nothing you have to do aside from celebrate in how free your accomplice feels to give up with you sincerely.

To encounter how thinking about sexual vitality can improve your sex life, attempt the accompanying activity alone or with an accomplice. It takes climax past the short form of "it feels so great and it's finished" to a degree of expanded thoughtful joy.

Conquering Your Fear of Letting Go

If you need to give up during sex yet something is keeping you down, it's basic to inspect and mend fears that can undermine your pleasure. Check whether the accompanying feelings of trepidation are halting you.

Regular Fears of Letting Go

1. Dread of losing control.

2. Dread of not performing.

3. Dread of taking too long to even think about having a climax.

4. Dread of talking your requirements.

5. Dread of agony, surrender, or passionate mischief.

6. Dread of losing yourself in a sweetheart.

7. Dread of getting fixated or excessively connected to a sweetheart.

To give up these feelings of dread, imagine another worldview of sexual vitality achievement. Get rid of old thoughts and grasp more genuine ones. The main switch is to for all time resign the thought that great sex is compared uniquely with execution. The conviction that "I'm not a genuine man or lady if I don't perform on order with an erection or a climax" is out of date and profoundly oblivious. It's horrid when sex is diminished to a challenge to continue substantiating yourself by how you perform—inspirations that additionally apply, pitiful to state, to prevailing in corporate America. This prompts execution nervousness, which just forestalls great sex and climaxes.

Similarly as attempting to nod off doesn't work, attempting to perform is damned. Do you think b-ball genius LeBron James is stressing over his exhibition when he's going for a sure thing? Or on the other hand Aretha Franklin when she's belting out a melody? Or then again Steve Jobs when he was concocting the iPad? I kindly question it. The equivalent goes for sex. Consideration ought to be centered around giving and accepting joy, not on desires for erections and climaxes. I encourage couples to be progressively real to life, increasingly inventive, all the more ready to address and impact separated thoughts that are against energy and hostile to adore.

Enthusiastic injuries can likewise prevent you from giving up. Lovemaking may trigger old damages, dread of surrender, or injury. When this happens to my patients, their first nature is often to close down. In psychoanalyst Alice Miller's enlightening book The Body Never Lies, she portrays the long haul outcomes of youngster maltreatment in the body, for example, ceaseless torment, deadness, and feebleness. Injury stops in our muscles and tissues until it's permitted to be discharged. One of my patients who battled with low confidence went through 10 years in a harsh marriage. She let me know, "My better half was into engaging in sexual relations during business breaks when we stared at the TV. He'd be done when Monday Night Football returned on. I would not like to make him frantic, so I faked climaxes." On those events, my patient loathed her significant other, herself, and the sex. No big surprise she experienced ceaseless pelvic torment. She adored her better half, however he was harming her with his damaging treatment and certainly not cherishing her the manner in which she had the right to be loved. My thumped persistent had arrived at that purpose of give up. At long last she was prepared to give up. During our treatment, she picked up the fortitude to leave the marriage and in the long run her pelvic agony vanished.

Systems that profited my patient and will help other people mend injury incorporate psychotherapy, bodywork, for example, vitality recuperating and back rub—and otherworldly work concentrating on self-empathy and the convoluted subject of absolution. If you have a past filled with injury that keeps you from giving up, I prescribe connecting with an advisor or manual for assist you with discharging it. As mending happens—and it will—giving up during lovemaking will feel more secure and the sexual vitality will turn out to be progressively pleasurable.

Maybe you keep away from giving up during sex because you're anxious about losing yourself in an accomplice or sacrificing your capacity. Like a few patients I've worked with, you may think that its difficult to remain revolved around sexual vitality. You may oppose the blending that occurs during climax because it causes you to feel imperceptible or expended. Incomprehensibly, you should be certain about what your identity is so as to appreciate such significant giving up. In any case the blissful disintegration of the sense of self during lovemaking may appear to be undermining. One undergrad enlightened me regarding her tangled feelings: "It feels like I part with my capacity when I let go. My beau causes me to feel so astounding, I'm apprehensive he'll have a piece of me that I'll never get back. Be that as it may, I'd successfully keep him." This addresses that it is so natural to get enticed by ecstasy, what individuals are enticed to surrender for it. Since Adam and Eve, sexual delight has made even the most reasonable individuals neglect their needs.

A related viewpoint is when one individual from a couple also significantly subordinates their character while thinking about a life partner or kids. What's been valuable for my patients right now to make a day by day life with increasingly singular significance and furthermore to define more clear limits. Possibly that implies coming back to class, accomplishing noble cause work, or demanding private time to ponder and seek after otherworldliness. If this sounds natural to you, as you pastor to your own needs you'll feel increasingly focused. Then it will be more secure to appreciate the opportunity of giving up, both during sexual vitality trades and in your relationship

Exercise: Orgasmic Meditation

Unwind and loosen up. Put aside some an opportunity to be erotic. Mood killer the telephone. Put a Do Not Disturb sign on your entryway. It's significant not to be hurried. To loosen up, take a couple of full breaths. Feel your midsection ascend with each in-breath, become gentler with each out-breath. Concentrate on the exotic nature of your body.

Have a climax. Stroke yourself. Enjoy a sexy idea. Excite each other with foreplay if you're with an accomplice. In the manner you like, regardless of whether you're self-pleasuring or having intercourse, carry yourself to climax.

Feel the climax rise, then pinnacle, then detonate. Let yourself dissolve into it. Give up to the joy.

Ponder. A brilliant method to feel sexual vitality move is to reflect following a climax. A moment or so following peak, sit in an upstanding position. It's a lot simpler to think when you're loose. Close your eyes: this intensifies any understanding. Breathe in and breathe out gradually. Concentrate daintily on the waiting euphoria of climax. Let it spread all through your body. Try not to drive anything. Sexual vitality travels through you normally. Give up to the sensations as they elevate. Relish the glow, shivers, or surge. Eyes despite everything shut, you may slip into a condition of natural mindfulness. You may see hues, vibrate from head to toe, or even feel God. Unconstrained instincts about individuals, work, or wellbeing may streak through. Afterward, make certain to compose these down and follow up on them. There is no time limit for this contemplation. Proceed as long as you prefer. Let the orgasmic vitality transport you to higher conditions of awareness, dreams, and joy.

The Difference Between Bonding and Overly Attaching to a Partner: Liberate Your Love

Holding with an accomplice is a characteristic piece of finding a good pace and of beginning to look all starry eyed at. In any case, getting excessively connected goes past sound sexual vitality trades and holding and is impairing. When you really love somebody, you're not keen on having the individual or keeping the person in question in your grasp because you're apprehensive about losing the relationship. Rather, you regard your accomplice's self-governance and soul. You're not very ensnared; rather you're standing together one next to the other. Genuine closeness is constantly a harmony among holding and giving up so the relationship can relax.

Take the accompanying test to decide your holding designs.

Test: Are You Overly Attached to a Partner?

1. Do you stick to your accomplice?

2. Would you like to have that person?

3. Is it accurate to say that you are often terrified of being relinquished or deceived?

4. Do you get restless when you don't get notification from the person in question each day if you're dating?

5. Do you continually consider the individual?

6. Do you begin fixating on an accomplice after you engage in sexual relations?

7. Does your accomplice feel you are attempting to control or choke out that person?

8. Do you believe you can't survive without the individual?

If you addressed yes to six to eight inquiries, you are amazingly excessively connected. Three to five yeses demonstrate that you are decently excessively joined. One to three yeses demonstrate that you tend to connect excessively. A score of zero demonstrates that you have sound holding with your accomplice.

A part of myself that I've gained ground in mending is my inclination to get excessively joined to men. During sex I bond rapidly and intertwine with a man, however I can't unfuse with him later. I begin longing for him and contemplating him continually. A portion of this is natural and beautiful yet turning out to be excessively appended crosses a line. I can get fixated and strongly hungry for contact, especially if I've been single for some time. I am a sexual being so if I haven't engaged in sexual relations for some time, I can get penniless. Being right now me (and numerous ladies) helpless against getting excessively joined. For example, if I don't get notification from the man for a couple of days, I can get on edge and scared of losing him or of being deserted. It's bad for me, and additionally, most men don't value this sort of reaction. So in my tantric sexual vitality meetings and in treatment, I found how to appreciate enthusiasm from a more grounded place. Here's the ticket:

1. I discovered that over-converging with a sexual accomplice can diminish sexual vitality charge. It really can be increasingly sexual to go all through serious association with an accomplice as opposed to continuing it. This gives the two sweethearts their space and all the more breathing room.

2. I don't "root" in a man. I root basically in myself and the earth. One way I do this when lovemaking is to picture my body forming roots into the dirt like a tree. I'm despite everything gave up to and inundated in delight, however I additionally keep a more full feeling of myself unblemished. I'm ready to isolate from him and all the more serenely consider us to be independent creatures.

3. In the wake of lovemaking, I think that its helpful to ponder with my accomplice and afterward state to one another, "I worship you. I respect you. I discharge you." This is a solid method to bond and delivers a beautiful harmony of adoring.

The answer for turning out to be excessively joined is to concentrate on strengthening your confidence while tending to and discharging fears, including the dread of deserting, which can make the need stick. Working with a talented relationship specialist or mentor can be profitable. These will assist you with creating self-governance and establishing. Being happy to give up the propensity to get excessively joined for a more advantageous bond will permit you to have progressively euphoric and pleasurable connections and sexual vitality trades without the torment of fixation.

Give up to Bliss

The objective of sexual vitality give up is to continue giving up in sound, positive ways, at your own pace, voluntarily. Lovemaking is a progressing give up to delight. What is euphoria? The word reference characterizes it as outrageous bliss, euphoria, and the delight of paradise. From my perspective, it's additionally the euphoria of associating with the body, to an accomplice, and to God. For me, this is where incredible streams merge, the convergence of human life and paradise. Delight isn't as removed as you would might suspect. It's in every case directly before us, at this time, when we can open to it.

Scholar Alan Watts stated, "When you are enamored with somebody, you do without a doubt consider them to be a celestial being." This "aha" minute can raise lovemaking from the physical to the otherworldly. Keep in mind: that perfect being you are having intercourse with is a similar individual who neglected to pay the lease a month ago and who in some cases doesn't do the dishes. Seeing the godlikeness in your accomplice while having intercourse, and consistently, is recognizing the phenomenal in the conventional. That is the key to rapture.

POSITIONS FOR SOFT PENETRATION

Because we as a whole merit a sound, glad sex life.

When it comes to engaging in sexual relations, I am everlastingly appreciative that I am a lady. For a certain something, I'm almost certain having a penis would occupy me tremendously. For something else, I don't need to stress over stuff like penis size, nor do I should be worried about the authentic Voldemort of having a penis: erectile brokenness.

For heaps of men, erectile brokenness corrupts (LOL, I said pollute, no opportunity to snicker about it now) all of their sexual connections. If they lose their erection during sex, they can feel flattened on something beyond the penis level. If they figure out how to keep their erection, all the enjoyment of engaging in sexual relations could be destroyed away by continually agonizing over to what extent this ol' erection will be hanging out.

While the different causes and solutions for erectile brokenness are one of a kind and often best treated with the assistance of a specialist, there is something you folks can attempt together: sex positions. Truth is stranger than fiction, relieving his erectile brokenness may be as simple as exchanging up your sex positions. Here are only a couple of my top picks that are similarly as enjoyment as they are therapeudic!

1. Cowgirl!

Man, I feel like the cowgirl sex position is the fix the entirety of the sex-having world, and I love it. For hell's sake, what's not to cherish? When you're on top, you set the speed, you control the weight, and you can turn into considerably more receptive to when and if he's going to pop. If he was on top he probably won't have the option to support himself, however with you at the reins (figuratively speaking) you can stop that clamor level.

2. Change that teacher!

Minister is super misjudged for a ton of reasons. If you aren't having some good times doing evangelist you're treating it terribly. It assists with erectile brokenness if you do it oppositely so his penis is entering you at a 90-degree point. Engaging in sexual relations thusly sort of changes the top side of his penis into the dildo from paradise. If they even make dildos in paradise. Proceeding onward. You'll get extra clitoral incitement, and he will have the option to last somewhat longer with this balanced style of entrance.

3. Spoon him!

Spooning isn't my preferred sex position because the degree of infiltration is so shallow. In any case, when it comes to sex positions for erectile brokenness, the shallowness of the entrance is the thing that you WANT. He won't be as invigorated as he may be utilizing other sex positions, which could assist him with keeping that penis up and dynamic throughout the night. In addition spooning = more nestles! The entirety OF THE CUDDLES! Thunder! (I just truly like snuggling).

4. Oral!

Prepare to be blown away. Now and again no measure of wonderful sex positions is going to stop the issue of erectile brokenness. In any case, that doesn't mean both of you have to abandon having a functioning and sound sex life. Sex positions aren't only constantly about a penis and vagina grinding away. Sex can be about your mouth as well, so don't keep it separate from the condition. If he is having a hard (or not all that hard) time getting his penis to take care of business, his mouth will work fine and dandy.

WHAT'S SO GOOD ABOUT PENETRATING DEEP?

There are two touchy zones profound inside the vagina that you or your accomplice might have the option to animate if you're not scared of a bit of spelunking.

One is the A-spot, which is situated along the front mass of the vagina close to the cervix. A few ladies report having the option to climax from A-spot incitement.

The subsequent spot is situated in a comparable situation along the back mass of the vaginal waterway, close to the butt-centric divider. Look at this guide with a picture to see it's definite area.

The A-spot is particularly known for not turning out to be overly sensitive after a climax, which implies that you may have the option to continue getting a charge out of penetrative sex or play time without the recoiling and uneasiness that can happen when you attempt to invigorate your G-spot or clitoris following cumming or squirting!

My most impressive sex deceives and tips aren't on this site. If you need to get to them and give your darling back-curving, toe-twisting, shouting climaxes that will keep them sexually fixated on you, then you can get familiar with these mystery sex procedures in my private and cautious pamphlet. You'll likewise get familiar with the 5 perilous missteps that will demolish your sex life and relationship. Get it here.

For what reason DO I SOMETIMES LIKE DEEP THRUSTING AND HATE IT OTHER TIMES?

As a lady, you may find that you now and then like profound entrance and aversion it at different occasions. This might be because of the situation of your cervix, which changes through an ordinary menstrual cycle. For instance, your cervix may be lower and increasingly open during your period and marginally after. The cervix is additionally harder during these occasions, which may make it increasingly helpless to torment from profound infiltration.

Then again, cervixes will in general raise and soften preceding ovulation and stay in that position during ovulation. This can make profound infiltration increasingly agreeable. Once in a while, a cervix can turn out to be so delicate and high during ovulation that it "mixes" in with the remainder of your vagina, which may be the ideal time to attempt profound infiltration.

Despite your cervical position and hardness, you probably won't appreciate the sentiment of a chicken – or dildo – pummeling into you if it's done too generally. Because your accomplice needs to dive deep, doesn't mean he needs to do it with power. Truth be told, further pushes may feel better with less power, so urge your accomplice to back off, which additionally gives you two time to appreciate it more. Also, you can without much of a stretch modify your own pace when stroking off.

If your accomplice is particularly blessed by the gods, it may appear that you can't keep away from profound infiltration, and sex may even be agonizing (more on that right now). Agonizing sex is known as dyspareunia and is more typical in ladies than men [2]. In any case, you can find a way to help forestall torment during sex.

Empower a lot of foreplay so your body is increasingly responsive to infiltration.

Use oil to ease inclusion and pushing.

Utilize a rooster ring or fold your fingers over your accomplice's penis to forestall profound pushing. More data here.

Engage in sexual relations in positions, for example, spooning or lady on-top where profound pushes are more uncertain or when you can control the speed and profundity of his penis in your vagina.

In any case, cervical incitement can be urgent for climax in certain ladies. Find out about cervical climaxes and how to have them.

Step by step instructions to GET MORE OUT OF DEEP PENETRATION

In any case, if you're a devotee of profound pushing, you'll need to have intercourse in all the enjoyment places that do empower you to feel your accomplice all the more profoundly. These can incorporate preacher, contingent on how your bodies coordinate, and doggy style. Correspondingly, because you can control profundity and speed during cowgirl, this may be your go-to position so you can feel every last bit of your accomplice within you!

Include PILLOWS

Cushions are an extraordinary method to accomplish profound infiltration for normal positions like evangelist. If you place one under your hips (butt or abs, contingent upon position), it raises them to make profound infiltration simpler. While a normal cushion can work after all other options have been exhausted, pads made of flexible foam are far and away superior because they don't pack. A few organizations, including Liberator, make pads of this material specifically for sex.

You can likewise have a go at hanging over or against other furniture in your home if the best doesn't help with profound infiltration. You may have a hassock that is actually the correct stature for Doggy or Turtle position, for instance.

Attempt TOYS

When it comes to toys, profound pushing is much simpler. There are penis extenders that your sweetheart can wear during sex to cause him to feel thicker and more. Notwithstanding, this is a sensitive issue to approach with any man as your accomplice would have an emptied inner self if you recommend that his normal life systems isn't exactly cutting it.

You can facilitate the discussion by advising him that you appreciate sex with him and appreciate sex in an assortment of ways. For most ladies who like profound infiltration, it may be charming, yet it would barely be a major issue. Guarantee that your accomplice knows this going into the discussion. If you're totally uncertain about his potential reaction, you can raise the possibility of these extenders or in any event, utilizing toys by clarifying that it's something you unearthed on the web – even point him to this book!

Luckily, there are various toys that he can use on you or that you can use without anyone else to accomplish the profundity that you like. Truth be told, there are such a large number of dildos and vibrators to name. Twofold dildos are normally somewhat more, yet you can utilize that length furthering your potential benefit to accomplish infiltration as profound as you can imagine it. Get familiar with dildos here.

Lady's Slim dildo offers seven creeps of entrance. You can likewise attempt the hardened steel Eleven by Njoy or a more drawn out glass dildo.

Furthermore, there are a lot of vibrators that are somewhere in the range of six and nine inches in length. Vibrators will in general have shorter insertable lengths, yet some G-spotters are particularly long, Fun Factory's Boss vibrators and the Ovo E8 are both somewhat longer than common.. Bunny vibes are often very huge, so you'll get both the size and profundity that you love.

In any case, you may have the option to accomplish profound pushes the manner in which you like even with a customary toy from your assortment.

Third Book: 101 SEX POSITIONS

Introduction

For any healthy relationship to prosper, the couple must indulge in healthy sex. Sex isn't just one of the basic primal needs. But at the same time, it is the way to create a bond that strengthens the two people who are a part of it.

When we talk of sex, the kind of topic it encompasses is huge and wide. Not everyone gets to enjoy the best level of sex, which infers something that some of us miss out on. This book aspires to help you reconnect with your inner sexual drive. Learn the best ways by which you can maximize your sexual potential and live every fantasy.

With these expert tips, you are sure to find a difference in your bedroom life and as a couple; you are much more likely to grow. The physical attraction you feel is a very strong component in any relationship, and as long as you don't feel the need to delight each other, the sparks won't fly.

So, it is time to shed all inhibitions as far as getting intimate is concerned. This book isn't meant solely for reading purposes. It will take you on a ride which will unravel the different layers of your body and help you understand your true sexual drive.

Sex isn't just about ejaculation or experiencing an orgasm. There is so much more to it. There are positions that you can experiment with. If you want your relationship to stay young, you need to be wild in love. This is why most successful couples who are always snuggling even in old age are those who do not fail to experiment. Your age isn't a delimiter to the number of times you need to have sex. It should be based on the stamina of your body and how your body reacts to your partner.

So, if all these have been a cause of concern or even if you are just curious to know about how the right sex drive could trigger the much-needed change in your life, we are here with the right book you need to pick and read.

Every chapter is meant to be put into action rather than read once and forgotten.

So, are you all set to get started?

Chapter 1: How Active Is Your Sex Life?

Before we divulge into the different positions and ways to improve your sex drive, we first need to get your analysis right. First of all, you have to understand as to where you stand and measure how deep the water is.

It is important to know that sex isn't something that you can compare with others. Someone may be doing it three or even five times a day, while you may have sex once every three days. This is not the sign of the warning bell yet.

Ideally, we believe that when you truly love your partner and feel the need, indulging in sex daily shouldn't be difficult. That being said, it is normal if the frequency is higher or lower.

So, here are a few things you should try and note down and then analyze your sex drive.

- How frequently do you have sex on average?
- If it is higher than the average, what do you think is the primary cause that triggers you?
- If your frequency is lower than normal, what do you feel is lacking in your relationship?
- Do you indulge in hot, passionate sex or is it mostly mild and soft?
- What factors are the most important to you when you want to have sex?
- Do you enjoy sex when the other person initiates it?
- Do you feel there has been a drop in the sex drive with your rising age graph?
- Do you love to experiment with new things when it comes to sex?

Note down the answers for each of them and you are likely to see a pattern. We are not going to dissect every single answer for you simply because every individual may have their interpretations of it.

These answers bother you solely and it is important to understand your primal needs. If you feel that your sex drive has weakened with age, there is nothing too wrong with it. However, what you need to do is to try and feel young again. Remember, age truly is nothing but a number. A man in his sixties could still be in his prime if he let himself believe so. George Clooney doesn't seem to be complaining about his age and neither is his wife!

Similarly, if you love mild and soft sex; it is alright, but once in a while, you need to experiment with the hot passionate kind where you can barely have your hands to yourself. This is because sex, when done in a routine, tends to get boring and loses its charm. You have to experiment, change, and bring in something dynamic to the table. Those of you who tend to be the wild, passionate one; you should try and go for soft and mild sex once in a while. Take your time slowly kissing your girl and caress her body before even starting with the foreplay. These little changes are what make your sexual drive all the more exciting.

So, each of these answers is important in helping you make a profile for yourself. By the end of the book, we are sure that you will witness some changes and want you to come back to this chapter and re-answer these questions. Then, it is time to play compare and contrast and you would be able to realize whether or not the book has been of any help to you.

Chapter 6: Anal Sex

Whenever there is a discussion of sex, anal sex often comes up. It is a little in the experimental category and almost each of us has tried our hand at it at least once. The thing about anal sex is that it can get painful and requires careful consideration of several parameters.

This is why we are going to have an elaborate discussion on the dynamic of anal sex and this will help you get a much better idea of how to do it.

The Guide to Anal Sex

Before we talk of some of the best positions and how you can make the most anal sex, it is important to know some precautions and set some ground rules. This is crucial because unlike the regular vagina sex, you need to exercise the right kind of caution.

Take the anal training before going the full way

We do not recommend starting anal sex unprepared. Remember, if you have never had anything in your anus, straight away asking for a penis to make way might not be the smartest of moves. The right thing to do is to experiment a little with small sex toys. This is important as it will stimulate and trigger the anal muscles and your body will be much better prepared to take in the penis. Do not create a fuss and be ready for a little anal training that can help you stay put for the big round of anal sex.

Have a thorough mutual discussion

Anal sex cannot be carried out if only one of the partners is willing. Remember, this is the kind of sex wherein both the parents need to have the same level of agreement. That being said, if during any time in between anal sex, any of the partners experience extra pain or discomfort, you should immediately stop having sex. Do not make things painful for each other. The idea is always to enjoy sex, have fun, and not make it look like a punishment.

The lube is mandatory

Always remember that there is a lot of difference between the vagina and the anus. The vagina has been so designed that it tends to self lubricate when aroused. However, the anus doesn’t work like that. So, if you do not want to bleed profusely and feel discomfort, the smart thing to do is to ensure that you use plenty of water-based lubes. Doing this can make the whole process smooth and much better for you. No matter how messy and dirty it gets, slather as much lube as needed and then go for the big penetration.

Steer clear of numbing creams

There are plenty of people who tend to choose numbing creams for the simple reason that it can take away the pain which is associated with anal sex. However, what you truly need to understand is that those creams can be potentially harmful in the long run.

When you use such numbing cream, your anus would be completely numb, so even if the penetration is too deep or there is an injury, you won't be able to feel and tell. This, in turn, could be the cause of several other problems. Until and unless you are willing to tolerate the pain, do not go for anal sex.

Try non-penetrative version first

When you are doing anal sex for the first time, you do not necessarily need to push the whole penis through. Remember, sex is more about the experience than the complete act of doing it. So, if you want to prepare your body and enjoy anal sex repeatedly, we want you to start slow. You could do things like fingering or oral sex, but do not get ahead with penetration.

This way, you prepare your body and your mind for what is likely to follow. After a few rounds of oral teasing, maybe in the next session, you could try penetrative sex. This will also prepare your anal muscles in a much better inner.

Never forget the condom

You absolutely must understand that there is no way you could do without the condom. When it comes to anal sex, the chances of transmitting STD and other infections are very high. This is why to ensure the safety of both the partners involved, make sure that the man is always wearing a condom. This is your primary line of defense which shouldn't be compromised at any cost whatsoever.

Foreplay is important

When it comes to anal sex, do not get started with penetration immediately. Like we have been emphasizing already; you have to engage in a fair deal of foreplay to prepare your body and anal muscles for the big event which will follow. There are plenty of foreplay and oral sex options that you could fiddle with and warm-up for the big session.

Maintain the basic hygiene

When we are dealing with anal sex, make sure to maintain the basic level of hygiene. This is why if you are using sex toys, keep them clean. Similarly, trim your nails and wash your hands before and after anal sex. Often, it is these little steps that ensure that you won't contaminate your body and you can prevent the transmission of bacterial borne diseases as well.

Once you are mindful of these factors, it will be relatively much easier and importantly safer to proceed with anal sex.

The Anal Sex Positions to Try

Let us see some of the best anal sex positions you can try to enjoy a great orgasm and satisfaction.

1. The Rear Entry

This is by far a popular choice for too many couples. It is like spooning but on the belly. The girl will need to lie down on her stomach, and she can spread her legs apart to give her man the ample amount of room to penetrate her.

The man needs to lie right on the top of his partner and face the same direction. After sufficient lubrication, he can then push his penis inside and give you the pleasure you have been seeking.

2. High Chair

This is one of the powerful anal sex positions which is likely to give you both a lot of thrill. The woman needs to sit on a chair so that the butt must stick out of it. The guy then needs to stand behind. He could kneel down or even squat based on the elevation of the chair.

The man would grab his partner's waist and slowly push his penis in the anus. The in and out moment is sure to feel like a rocking chair and will drive both of you crazy with passion.

3. The Leapfrog

This has a slight variation from the regular doggy style. When you perform this position, think similar to doggy style but make sure that your (woman's) chest rests on the bed. The extra elevation ensures that your man will get all the room to push him inside you.

Once again, have ample lubrication to make the whole process smooth and enjoyable.

4. The Turtle Position

This position is for those couples who like to play the submissive-dominant game. The woman needs to be on her knees and then pull them inside. This gives her hips an elevated arch and the man could kneel and draw her waist towards him before pushing his penis in the anus and giving her a fun-filled ride.

This position can be uncomfortable for the woman and you should be ready to improvise the moment you want to.

5. The Burning Man

Yet another position wherein the man achieves the dominant role and you could play the submissive lead.

The position is simple, but you would need a tabletop or even a sofa. The woman needs to lean on the top of the sofa or the table and bed so that her anal end is thrusting out. The man then spoons you from behind and after enjoying some oral sex, he pushes his cock inside your hole. It is important to ensure that your table or sofa is such that it doesn't hurt you when leaning on it. Keeping a pillow or a blanket might be a good alternative.

This form of anal sex has the potential to get rough as your man could do all he wishes since you are bent on the table and can only moan and shriek in pleasure and pain. So, for those who love rough sex, this is surely a good position to try.

6. The Pearly Gates

If you are looking for an anal sex position that could feel a little exciting, this is it. In this position, the man needs to lie down on his bed. He can spread apart his legs a little, but the feet should be fairly planted. The woman would now get on top of the man and face the same side. Make sure to position yourself in such a way that the man's penis could find the woman's butthole and he could slowly but steadily make an entry and please you thoroughly.

This position allows for a lot of cuddling, foreplay, and even fingering as well. So, feel free to elevate your senses before getting downright dirty and rough.

7. The Jockey Sex

Those women who love to have their men firmly in corner and make the most of this form of sex. Here, the woman needs to lie down and the legs don't even need to be spread apart.

The man would then approach you from the back and sit with his knees bent. He needs to lean right over the back and then he can get the best angle to push his penis inside your butthole and drive you crazy with his rocking to and fro movement.

So, these are some of the best anal sex positions which you can surely try. Remember, regardless of which position you choose, it is very important to observe the right rules which we had discussed earlier. Practicing safe sex is crucial to ensure that both the partners can benefit from it.

This is not the ultimate bible as there are endless other positions that you can try. Come up with anything out of your mind, the only rule is that never stop having fun!

If you are up for a round of anal sex, you could try some of these positions and like always, note down your experience. This will prepare you better for the best sex experience of all time.

Chapter 7: Sex Games and Role Play

How often do you engage in role-playing and what is your opinion about it? We believe that sex games and role play are excellent ways to improve the kind of sex life you are having simply because it creates a different kind of passion.

So, if you want to do something kinky and maybe experiment with games and role play, we recommend you be up for it. There are several kinds of challenges that you can throw at each other as this tends to rev up the excitement among the couples and gives them something new to hold on and explore as well.

So, let us talk of some of the possible sex games and then move on to the kind of role pay antics you could engage in.

The Striped Down Twister

We have all heard and played the classic board game twister. You have to play it the same way, the only difference is that every time someone fails, they have to remove a layer of clothing until someone strips completely and you can then move to the bed and take the game to a different level altogether.

Truth or Dare

Give the classic truth or dare a strip twist. The questions should all be related to sex or the sexual fantasy you have and the ones you have lived. When it comes to daring, have sex-related dares, it could be things like give me a blow job, strip for me, give me a lap dance, do pole dance or anything else. The only thing you need to remember here is that the game should be played with mutual consent and the boundaries should be well decided beforehand.

The Sex Dice

You could buy the sex dice from an adult store or make two sets of notes yourself. In one of them, you should jot down the name of the body parts and the other one; it should be the sexual actions you have to do.

One partner will take out the note from one set and the other from the next one. All you have to do is perform the action on the selected body part and thereby see who does what best. This is a great way to have fun in bed.

Of course, there are endless more games. Any board game can be turned into a sex game by giving it a strip angle. Every time you lose, you will have to remove one pair of clothing. Even challenge games could be turned to sex games by giving a sex-related dare at the end of the round.

So, make full use of your imagination and let sex be the torchbearer to the games to give you a fun-filled night.

Now that we are done with sex games, we will shift our focus to role play. If you haven't quite engaged in role-play, we want you to do so simply because once you enjoy the thrill, there is no way you will go back. The best thing about role play is that the sky is the imagination. You can do as much or as little as you please because there is absolutely no one to stop you whatsoever!

The Role-Play Sessions

Why should you do it?

When we are talking of role-play sessions, the very first thing which we are going to talk about is why you should at all engage in it. We have some clear reasons for you to do so.

☐ *Sets the momentum for the rest of the sexy night to follow*

☐ *It is a great way to spice things up*

☐ *Makes you feel different*

☐ *Helps partners come closer and are experimental*

☐ *Great way to keep sex fun*

☐ *Offers plenty of room to try new things*

So, now that the reasons are clear, we are now going to focus on some of the possible role-play ideas that will give you the incentive to try them tonight with your partner. Remember, the sky is the limit when it comes to these games and once you get a hang of it; you would have a hard time letting it go.

1. The Professor And Student

Who doesn't love a good college romance? We have all fantasized about one or the other of our teachers in schools and colleges where our hormones were always on a rage.

One of you could be a professor and make sure to wear a tie and glasses and strip the rest. This makes you a very sexy professor indeed; you could use a ruler in hand or even chalk to go with the image.

When the other one is dressed like a college girl, go for pigtails or even braided hair. You could wear red lipstick and wear a sexy school uniform.

Now, the student approaches the professor who scolds her for being a bad girl. In turn, she could request the professor to help her with her classes and she would do anything in return. Make sure to flash your cleavage or even your butt when you do so and he could spank your ass for being a bad girl again. Do what you please and create enough drama until both of you can barely hold it anymore! Then, jump on the bed and have the best class there!

2. The Boss And Employee

Once you are done with the college romance, why not head to the office room right away? Your man could be a mean boss and he could wear a coat and let go of the pants. The man needs to have a stern and strict voice.

The woman could dress like a regular employee or better she could just be wearing the heels and then for the scene, you could narrate things like, "Oops, I forgot my attire, will you let me off the hook, boss?"

The idea here is to have a desk and make each other horny. Try and hint at hot, angry sex and the employee could be submissive and the boss could play the dominant role.

3. The Doctor And Nurse

Who said hospitals can't be fun! You could play the role of a naughty, slutty nurse and a sleazy doctor whose hands end up slipping on the nurse's butt every time he wants to operate.

The scene can get downright sexy and you have the option to play it anyways. The nurse could complain about possible pain in her vagina and the doctor could finger her to see what is amiss.

Once again, it all comes down to your imagination and one thing is for sure, there is no denying that role-playing tends to be a lot of fun!

If you are looking to rev things in bed and you want an exciting sex life ahead of you, we recommend the right level of role-playing and sex games. These are the little things that are sure to bring about a change in your sex drive.

If you haven't ventured in these fields yet, we want you to do so now and see how it feels. There is a very strong possibility that you will love the experience and get hooked to it.

Chapter 8: Sex Toys

Do you use sex toys? How comfortable are you with buying sex accessories which can help you have an exciting bedroom life? You need to know that there is absolutely nothing wrong with using sex toys. Go to adult sex shops and explore the wide range of products available there. It will open your mind to a world of new possibilities.

Simultaneously, if you do not want to head anywhere, you could simply go to an online store and check out the vast available options. The idea is to open up to the possibility of using these toys and witnessing how it helps you feel the vibe.

So, here are some of the possible reasons as to why you should opt for sex toys.

Taking the pressure off

There is absolutely no doubt about the fact that using sex toys is sure to take off the pressure from both the partners. Women sometimes find it harder to orgasm and they may need external stimulation to reach their heightened level. In these cases, having the best sex toys could make things easier and pressure off your partner.

Whether or not a woman has experienced an orgasm isn't directly related to her partner's performance. So, feel free to use the best sex toys to forget the right kind of stimulation and thereby enjoy better orgasms.

Improved quality of sex

With the sex toys, you can explore your insides a lot more and this also creates a deeper and better level of sexual experience. Several women tried sex toys after much hesitation but enjoyed it a great deal on their first attempt. You may also get hooked to them. So, the idea simply is to be ready to explore and to try and seek the best kind of pleasure in it.

Try and involve your partner as much as you can as this will make for a hot, steamy, and passionate night.

You could make smart use of remote-controlled sex toys, remotely operated dildos, nipples clamps, handcuffs and more.

Mutual masturbation

Have you ever tried mutual masturbation? It is always known to be a massive turn on. When you both are using sex toys, you could sit together and use them to experience masturbation.

This is also advantageous because when you are masturbating in front of your partner, they will be able to see what it is that you like and what it is that turns you on. This information could be vital when you are engaging in sex later on.

Also, men are known to have a thing for watching women masturbate. So, when you use sex toys and push a dildo inside you and climax, your man will get real horny and take you on a long wild ride later.

Great way to live your sexual fantasies

We all have some steamy sexual fantasies that we want to turn to life. So, if you too have some deep, dark, and secret desires, you can try to make those turn true as well. The best way to make it happen is by buying sex toys that can help you live them and thereby enjoy your time to the fullest.

Feel free to play with your imagination and see how it kicks starts the journey of your sexual fantasy turning true.

Using together could help you bond

Many couples have felt that when they go out together to buy sex toys and accessories to spice up the sex game, it helps them bond better and come together. There are many different ways you could feel the heat and passion rise between the two of you, and choosing to buy sex toys might be one such way.

So, there are endless reasons for you to go ahead and buy sex toys. The key thing here is to indulge as much as you are comfortable. Remember, with your partner, there should be no apprehensions whatsoever and you should both be completely transparent with each other.

So, live every sexual fantasy and take things outside your primary zone by choosing to buy the right kind of sex toys and sex accessories. Go to a sex shop and see what they have got for you. Take some things home and experiment as much as you want with it. Every movement is sure to bring both of you closer and help you witness something remarkable.

So, if you are all set to revamp your sex life, one of the smart ways of doing it is by introducing sex toys in your life. You would be amazed at how vast this world is and how much you can foray into it. Buy things one at a time and when you seem hooked to the experience, go all out and buy things that excite the two of you.

Sex toys are known to bring about a massive change in the passion level as they bring in a new dimension to the already existing one. Even when you feel that passion seems to be going out a little, with the right sex toys, you might be able to infuse it one more time. It is all about experimenting and enjoying what the experiment has to offer.

Make sure you try and venture in this territory and note down how good or surreal the whole experience felt. Always be vocal with your partner. Remember that you both should be on the same page. The moment any of you feel uncomfortable, you should stop using immediately because sex is never about forcing your choices on your partner. It has to be mutual consent and agreement as it is only then that the real fun starts to kick in.

Chapter 10: 101 Positions

Man Trap

This is a variation of the missionary position. The female should lie back on a bed in the missionary position and have the male lay on top. As he begins to thrust, the female can wrap her legs around him and control the speed and pace of sex.

This is great if you just want some simple sex. You can put little twists on the move like arching the back for better stimulation. Wrapping the legs around the male will also get him going a lot faster!

1. The female should lie on her back in the missionary position – legs open wide and slightly bent.

2. The male should position himself over the female and face her.

3. The male can then penetrate the vagina, just as in the ordinary missionary position.

4. As the male begins thrusting, or when it feels best, the female can wrap her legs around the male and 'trap' him, forcing him closer of allowing some extra room for him to re-position.

5. Tip: Using a pillow under the female's back can help cause an arch. This will greatly increase pleasure and make things much more comfortable when wrapping her legs around the male.

Safety Tips

This position can strain the female's lower back, so make sure support is provided by using a pillow or cushion! Be sure to ask whether your partner is comfortable and not in any pain at any point and don't be ashamed if you need to say something because you are uncomfortable!

The Deckchair

The male should sit on the bed with his legs stretched out and his hands behind him to support his weight. He should lean back and bend his elbows slightly. The female should lie back on a pillow facing him and put her feet up on to his shoulders. She can then move her hips forwards and back and begin having sex.

This is an amazing position for very deep penetration for G-spot stimulation.

1. The male should sit on a bed with his legs stretched out. He can use his hands behind him to support his weight.
2. He should then carefully lean back and bend his elbows slightly for further support and control.
3. The female should then position herself by the male's feet, facing him and laying back on a pillow for support.
4. Once in position, the female can begin moving closer to the male until her feet are up on his shoulders.
5. Finally, she can move her hips towards his penis for insertion.
6. In this position, once penetrated, it is best for the female to be in control and thrust her hips back and forth to get the best control and stimulation.

Safety Tips

This position can cause a lot of strain on the female's lower back, so make sure support is provided by using a pillow or cushion! Be sure to ask whether your partner is comfortable and not in any pain at any point and don't be ashamed if you need to say something because you are uncomfortable!

Corridor Cosy

This one can be tricky as you need to be in an enclosed area. The male needs to lean against a wall and shuffle his way towards the floor until his feet touch an opposing wall. The female should climb down on top of his legs, supporting her weight. Her legs should be left dangling and she can begin thrusting.

This is a great one for adventurous and exciting sex!

1. Find an enclosed area with secure structures such as a thin corridor, hallway, or other appropriate settings.

2. The male should lean against one side of the wall and lower himself carefully by extending his legs outwards to the opposing wall.

3. IMPORTANT: The male's feet should always remain on the floor and securely in place at the base of the opposing wall.

4. The female should position herself on top of him and face towards him.

5. The female can begin lowering herself towards the penis for penetration, using either the walls around her or the male's shoulders for support. The female's legs should be left dangling while she is on top.

6. Finally, she can begin thrusting back and forth.

7. Tip: If this position is too taxing on the strength of either the male or the female, consider having the male position himself in a lower position so that the female's legs can reach the floor. She can then use her legs to help support her weight.

Safety Tips

The male needs to make sure that he can support his partner's weight and that he isn't going to slip and fall to the floor completely. Likewise, the female should support her weight as best she can to avoid potential injury.

Twister Stalemate

The female should begin by laying on her back with her legs apart. Her partner should kneel on all fours in between her legs. The female should then lift herself, wrapping her arms around his chest for support. She should then slowly bring up her legs so her feet are flat on the bed.

This is a great position for deep penetration and stimulating the G-spot!

1. The female should lie down on her back with her legs apart and slightly bent at the knee.

2. The male should then position himself in-between her legs, facing her and on all fours i.e. on his hands and feet.

3. The female should then wrap her arms up around the male's chest for support. This will require some strength from the female.

4. The female can then bend her legs and begin to raise her hips. Her feet should now be flat on the bed.

5. Finally, she can guide the penis into her vagina for penetration.

Safety Tips

This position requires some upper body strength from the female. She should make sure to be holding on tightly to her partner as he thrusts.

The Spider

You should start by facing each other. The female should climb on to her partner's lap and allow penetration. Her legs should be bent on either side of him and the male should be doing the same. The female should lay back first, slowly followed by the male, until both heads are on the bed. Now, move slowly and calmly.

This is a great one for slow sex to enhance stimulation before trying to reach climax – a good one if you have a lot of time.

1. Both the male and female should begin by sitting on a bed and facing towards each other.

2. The female should then shuffle forward and sit on her partner's lap.

3. This is the point where penetration should occur. The female must remain on top of her partner's lap.

4. Once penetrated, the female should slowly lean backwards and bend her back until her head is on the bed. Her arms can then be positioned outwards until comfortable.

5. The male should repeat this stage, leaning back slowly until his head is on the bed.

6. The female can then begin thrusting forwards and backwards.

Safety Tips

This position requires penile flexibility, else there is a risk of the male straining his suspensory ligaments!

If you want to find out if the male's penis is flexible enough, have him stand against a wall. Pull his penis gradually down. If the penis can point directly down to the ground without causing pain then you should be fine to perform this position, but still be careful.

The female should stay still when the male is initially penetrating her and guide the penis to the vagina. The female should wait while he finds the most comfortable position and angle to thrust without injury.

Speed Bump

The female should lay on her stomach and spread her legs. The male should then enter from behind.

The benefit of this position is that things can heat up and speed up very quickly. It is a great position for getting a little rough or if you're having a quickie!

1. The female should lay down on her stomach and spread her legs as wide as she can while remaining comfortable.

2. The male should position himself on top of the female to penetrate from behind, both facing the same way.

3. Once in the position, the male should use his arms to support his weight while he guides his penis towards her vagina for penetration.

4. Finally, the male can perform upwards and downwards thrusts.

Safety Tips

This position can cause a lot of strain on the female's lower back, so make sure support is provided by using a pillow or cushion! Be sure to ask whether your partner is comfortable and not in any pain at any point and don't be ashamed if you need to say something because you are uncomfortable!

Triumph Arch

The male should sit down with his legs stretched out straight. The female should straddle him with her legs either side and kneel over his penis. Once she has been penetrated, she can lean back until laying down on his legs.

This position can give the female a great orgasm and the male can stimulate her clitoris during sex.

1. The male should sit down on a bed with his legs stretched out and straight.

2. The female should straddle over the male, bending her knees until over his penis.

3. Once in position and penetrated, the female can slowly lean back until she is laying down on his legs.

Safety Tips

This position requires penile flexibility, else there is a risk of the male straining his suspensory ligaments!

If you want to find out if the male's penis is flexible enough, have him stand against a wall. Pull his penis gradually down. If the penis can point directly down to the ground without causing pain then you should be fine to perform this position, but still be careful.

The female should stay still when the male is initially penetrating her and guide the penis to the vagina. The female should wait while he finds the most comfortable position and angle to thrust without injury.

The Standing Wheelbarrow

For this position, begin in the doggy style position and have the female rest her forearms on some pillows. Her partner should kneel behind her with one knee bent up to keep himself steady. Once he has penetrated, he should hold her legs and slowly lift her as he stands.

This position is great if you are just experimenting and just having fun! Otherwise, it is a bit difficult and isn't very well rated for sensation.

1. The female should begin on her hand and knees, facing away from the male (the doggy style position).

2. The female can lean her upper body down towards the floor and rest her forearms on a pillow.

3. The male should kneel behind her with one knee bent for extra support.

4. He can then position himself towards her for penetration from behind.

5. Finally, the male should grab hold of the female's legs, wherever comfortable and secure, and support her weight as he carefully raises to a standing position.

6. He can then thrust forward and back.

Safety Tips

The male should keep his knees slightly bent when thrusting. If either of you feels uncomfortable during the position, you should let the other know and try something else! This one isn't for you.

Sultry Saddle

In this position, the male lays down on his back with his legs bent and apart – the standard position when the male is on the bottom. The female should slide herself between his legs, almost at a right angle to his body. For support, one hand should be placed on his chest, the other on his leg.

This position relies on the female rocking back and forth until she can feel him hitting her G-spot. The great thing about this position is that the female is completely in control, so it is one of the better if G-spot stimulation is what you need to reach an orgasm.

1. The male should lie down on a bed on his back, facing upwards. His legs should be bent at the knee and apart.

2. The female should position herself over the male on her feet or knees, whichever is most comfortable.

3. She can then lower herself to allow for penetration.

4. Once penetrated, the female should place one hand on the male's leg, and the other on his chest for support. She can then use these supports to help her thrust and control her stimulation.

Safety Tips

This position can strain the female's lower back, so make sure support is provided by using a pillow or cushion! Be sure to ask whether your partner is comfortable and not in any pain at any point and don't be ashamed if you need to say something because you are uncomfortable!

The Propeller

The female should lay on her back with her legs straight and together. The male should lie down on top but be facing down towards her feet. Once penetrated, the male should make small motions with his hips instead of thrusting.

This is a very difficult position and takes some practice to master!

1. The female should lie on her back with her legs straight and together.

2. The male should position himself on top of her in the 180-missionary position i.e. over the female but be facing her feet. He should, as usual, be using his arms for support to hold his body weight.

3. The male can then shuffle backwards until he can penetrate the female.

4. Once penetrated, rather than thrusting back and forth, the male should rotate his hips in small circular motions in a 'propeller'-like movement.

Safety Tips

This position requires penile flexibility, else there is a risk of the male straining his suspensory ligaments!

If you want to find out if the male's penis is flexible enough, have him stand against a wall. Pull his penis gradually down. If the penis can point directly down to the ground without causing pain then you should be fine to perform this position, but still be careful.

The female should stay still when the male is initially penetrating her and guide the penis to the vagina. The female should wait while he finds the most comfortable position and angle to thrust without injury.

The Lustful Leg

Start by standing close and facing each other. The female should have one leg on the bed and the other on top of the male's shoulder, while wrapping her arms around his back and neck. Then he should carefully penetrate.

Once in position, this is a great move that feels fantastic! It does, however, require some endurance.

1. Both the male and female should begin by standing up beside a bed and facing one another.

2. The female should wrap her arms around the male's neck and shoulders for support.

3. The female can then raise one leg on to the edge of the bed. The other leg can then be raised to the male's shoulder.

4. Once in position, penetration can take place.

Safety Tips

This position requires penile flexibility to avoid the risk of the male straining his suspensory ligaments!

If you want to find out if the male's penis is flexible enough, have him stand against a wall. Pull his penis gradually down. If the penis can point directly down to the ground without causing pain then you should be fine to perform this position, but still be careful.

The female should stay still when the male is initially penetrating her and guide the penis to the vagina. The female should wait while he finds the most comfortable position and angle to thrust without injury.

The Waterfall

The male should sit in a sturdy chair. The female can then climb on top with her legs either side of him. She should lean back until her head is on the floor.

The clitoris is very accessible in this position so is great for stimulation during sex. There is also a lot of friction inside the vagina so this is a great all-rounder for reaching orgasm.

1. The male should find a secure chair and sit on it.

2. The female can then position herself facing towards the male with her legs either side of him.

3. The female should then lower herself on to his penis for penetration.

4. Once inserted, the male should use his hands to support the female behind her back and bottom.

5. The female should then slowly lean backwards until her head is on the floor.

6. While performing step 5 above, the male should take care to support the female's weight however necessary, and the female should take care to move slowly to ensure that the male is not experiencing any strain or discomfort.

Safety Tips

This position requires penile flexibility, else there is a risk of the male straining his suspensory ligaments!

If you want to find out if the male's penis is flexible enough, have him stand against a wall. Pull his penis gradually down. If the penis can point directly down to the ground without causing pain then you should be fine to perform this position, but still be careful.

The female should stay still when the male is initially penetrating her and guide the penis to the vagina. The female should wait while he finds the most comfortable position and angle to thrust without injury.

A pillow should also be used on the floor to comfort the female's head during sex.

The Challenge

This is a difficult position (hence the name) and shouldn't be attempted unless you are confident and have tried lots of different positions before – it requires strength and flexibility.

The female should stand on a chair and bend her knees until in the sitting position. She should lean forward with her elbows on her knees. The male should then enter her from behind.

This one is hard to master. If it is too hard for you, you could also have the female simply stand on the ground and lean forward on to a chair as shown in the illustration below.

1. A sturdy and secure chair should be found for this position. It may be useful for the chair to be against a wall.

2. The female should mount the chair and stand up, facing towards the back of the chair and away from the male.

3. She should then carefully bend her knees until in a sitting position.

4. The female should then place her elbows on her knees, and hold on to the back of the chair with her hands.

5. Finally, once comfortably in position, the male should approach the female from behind for penetration.

Safety Tips

Make sure the chair is very sturdy and you have good footing. The male should support the female throughout and should have a firm hold of the female's waist to keep her steady.

The Supernova

For this position, the female should begin on top of the male on a bed or other comfortable place. The male should have his head near the edge. The female should place her feet either side of him and allow penetration by squatting down on his penis. She can then lean back on to her arms behind her.

The female should rock back and forth until she can feel herself reaching climax. When reaching climax, she should lean forward to her knees and shift the male's upper body off the edge of the bed until she reaches orgasm.

This position is all about timing, but if done right can be really fun and give a great orgasm.

1. The male should begin by lying down, facing upwards and with his knees slightly bent and apart. His head should be near the edge of the bed.

2. The female should place her feet on either side of the male's waist and squat down in a straddle position for penetration.

3. The female should then place her hands and arms behind her on the bed and lean backwards. Her arms should be locked and providing most of the support.

4. She can then begin thrusting back and forth.

5. When approaching orgasm, the female should launch her upper body forward and on to her knees. This should slightly shuffle the male's head and upper body off of the bed.

6. Tip: Ensure that the timing is right with the once – it might take some practice. But, once done correctly, this can lead to a fantastic orgasm.

Pirate's Bounty

This position is great when you and your partner want to go a bit more out there to reach orgasm. It allows for deep penetration and total clitoral stimulation so is amazingly efficient at getting you to an orgasm.

To get in this position, the female should lay down on her back and the male should kneel in front of her. She should place one leg on her partner's shoulder and the other around his thigh. A pillow can also be used under the female's back to provide support.

1. The female should lie on her back facing upwards towards the ceiling with her legs apart.

2. The male should kneel in front of her, facing towards her.

3. The female should place one leg up on the male's shoulder (whichever is most comfortable) and the other leg should remain beside his thigh.

4. A pillow should be placed under the female's back to provide support and place her in an arch to increase stimulation.

5. The male should then penetrate the female.

6. While having sex, either the male of the female can easily stimulate the clitoris for further stimulation. This is best done when the female is approaching orgasm.

Advanced Doggy Style

This is a simple variation of the traditional doggy style, but with a better chance of achieving an orgasm.

To do this, assume the normal doggy style position and guide the female's head until it is against the bed. Her back should be bent slightly with her bum in the air. Now, place a pillow or blanket under her stomach to rest on. Make sure the female is relaxed. Thrust downwards at a hard and steady pace for several minutes until she reaches orgasm.

1. Both the male and the female should assume the normal doggy style position - the female should be on her hands and knees, facing away from the male.

2. The female should allow for a slight inwards arch in her back i.e. she should raise her bottom and chest while allowing her stomach to arch inwards towards the bed.

3. A pillow or large blanket should be placed under the female's stomach for her to rest on and she can then lower her upper body closer to the surface of the bed.

4. Finally, the male can penetrate from behind.

5. The male should continuous thrust in a firm downwards motion at a steady pace of several minutes. His motion should become faster and harder as the female approaches orgasm.

G-Spot Missionary

Assume the normal missionary position. Then place the female's legs on to the male's shoulders. A pillow should be placed under her lower back for support and comfort. Slightly push forward until the female's bum lifts off the surface of the bed. Begin thrusting hard at a consistent pace. You can bring yourself closer to her to be more intimate or further away to thrust harder.

1. The female should lie down on her back, facing upwards with her knees slightly bent and legs apart. A pillow should be placed beneath the female's back to create an arch and provide support.

2. The male should position himself on top of the female, facing her and using his arms to support his body weight.

3. The male should penetrate the female just as he would in the ordinary missionary position.

4. Once inserted, the male should push forward (before thrusting) to slightly raise the female's bottom off the surface of the bed. The female's bottom should remain elevated from the surface of the bed throughout.

5. Finally, the male can begin thrusting at a constant and firm pace.

6. Throughout this position, the male can slow down his thrust and bring himself closer to the female for intimacy, and lift away from the female for harder and faster thrusts as she approaches orgasm.

Flatiron

The female should lie face down with her hips slightly elevated. A pillow should be used for support under her stomach. She should spread her legs out and straight. The male should mount her from behind with his legs on the outside of hers and penetrate. This position allows for easy access for anal sex or vaginal intercourse, but limits access to the clitoris so keep that in mind if you need clitoral stimulation.

1. The female should lie face down on a bed with her hips slightly elevated. Her legs should be comfortably apart.

2. A pillow should be placed under the female's stomach for support.

3. The female should now spread her legs further apart and keep them straight.

4. The male can then position himself on top of the female using his arms for support.

5. Once in position, the male can penetrate the female virginally or anally and begin thrusting. His legs should on the outside of the females, but they can remain on the inside if the male finds this uncomfortable.

6. The male is now in control and can build up to a hard thrust.

The Sunday Afternoon

This is a much easier position to try when you want to reach an orgasm. It's a great choice for easy access to the clitoris if you need clitoral stimulation to reach climax. It is a variation of an X position, like The Scissors.

The male begins laying on his side and the female on her back. She puts one leg over his outer-side hip and the other wrapped around his lower leg to pull him close. The male gently penetrates and begins thrusting upwards.

1. The male should lay down on his side beside the female. The female should begin by lying on her back.

2. The female should then place her outside leg over the outer-hip of the male. The other leg should then wrap around the male's lower leg. At the end of this movement, the female should transition from being on her back to being on her side, facing the male.

3. The female can then use her legs to bring the male in close and allow for penetration.

4. The male can then gently begin thrusting towards the female in an upwards motion.

Mastery

This is a version of the cowgirl position and doesn't ask for too much physical effort from either partner, but give the male easy access to the clitoris and the breasts for stimulation during intercourse.

The male and female should face each other in the cowgirl position, with the female seated on his lap. Her legs should be kneeling outside his. The position allows for couples to get close during sex and lean back for new sensations.

1. The male and female should assume the cowgirl position. This is achieved by the male lying on his back with his knees slightly bent and his legs slightly apart. The female can then straddle on top of the male's hips.

2. The female should transition so that she is in the same position, but resting on her knees rather than her feet.

3. The female should take control of allowing penetration by guiding the male's penis inside of her.

4. This position allows for a lot of variation depending on how the female is feeling during intercourse. She can lean forwards to come close to the male for intimacy, sit upwards for firmer thrusts or lean backwards using her arms for support when approaching orgasm for G-Spot stimulation.

5. When leaning back, the male also has very easy access to provide clitoral stimulation.

Scissors

This is an X position and can be a challenge for those not willing to commit to it. The female should lay down on her back and her partner should enter her from the sides – her clitoris should be up against his top leg.

1. The female should lie down on her back, facing the ceiling.

2. The female should ensure that her legs are open wide to allow access by the male.

3. The male should begin in a sideways position away from the female with his feet in the same place as the female's.

4. The male can then begin moving towards the female between her legs.

5. As the male approaches, the female should raise her back and bottom to allow the male's lower leg to be positioned underneath.

6. As the male shuffles closer to the vagina, the female should help by positioning herself closer to allow for penetration – the female's clitoris should be up against the male's outer leg's thigh.

7. Penetration can now take place.

8. Once both the male and female are comfortable, both can begin gently thrusting towards each other.

The Dirty Dangle

Begin by having the female lay down on her back at the foot end of the bed. Have the male mount on top in the missionary position. The female should start moving back little by little until her head, shoulders and arms flay off the back of the bed towards the floor. The excitement of this position can be a new experience for lots of people and encourage orgasm.

1. The female should lie down on her back at the foot end of a bed.

2. The male should mount on top of the female in the missionary position, using his arms to support his weight.

3. Once in position, the female should start shuffling slowly backwards until her head, shoulders and arms flay off the back of the bed towards the floor.

4. Both the male and female should support each other during the above movement to ensure both are secure.

5. The male can then penetrate and begin thrusting.

6. The increased blood flow to the female's head aims to provide a greater and more fulfilling orgasm. This can be done before or during intercourse.

Lazy Male

With this move, there is less thrusting involved and move up and down motions. There is lots of eye contact that can bring you closer to your partner and increase your chance of reaching an orgasm.

For this position, the male should prop his body up with some pillows against a wall or the bed's headboard. Here you can control the rhythm of sex. Have the female sit in the cowgirl position with her legs wrapped around his body and stay up and close.

1. The male should sit up against a wall or the headboard of a bed, using pillows for support.

2. The female should position herself above the male's hips and squat down to a straddle position.

3. The female can then transition into a kneeling straddle position and allow for penetration.

4. The female can then control the rhythm of intercourse as she begins thrusting up and down.

Face Off

Have the male sit down on the edge of the bed or sofa. The female should sit down on his lap, facing him. From here there should be a lot of friction on the clitoris which is great for reaching orgasm if you need direct clitoral stimulation to reach an orgasm.

1. The male should find a sturdy bed or sofa and sit towards the edge.

2. The female should position herself over him with her legs either side and lower herself down on to his lap facing him.

3. As the female lowers herself, she should reach a kneeling position with her legs either side of the male.

4. The female can then allow penetration by guiding the penis towards her vagina.

5. During this position, the female should thrust forwards to increase the friction on her clitoris and achieve the maximum stimulation.

The OM

For this position, have the male sit down with his legs crossed while the female sits on his lap, facing him. Next, the female should wrap her legs around him and his legs should be wrapped around the back of her, still crossed. Pull each other close together and rock back and forth. You should look each other in the eyes as you climax.

1. The male should sit down, either on a bed or the floor, with his legs crossed.

2. The female should position herself over the male and be facing towards him.

3. The female should wrap her legs around the back of the male's bottom and cross them over behind him.

4. Penetration can now take place.

5. Once penetration has been achieved, both males and females can pull each other close and rock and forth.

This is an intimate position and encourages both partners to remain close. The aim is to achieve good eye contact as the female approaches orgasm.

The Sea Shell

Have the female lay down on her back with her legs raised and out. The male should lie on his stomach on top and be facing her as he penetrates, just like the missionary. The female's legs should be far apart to allow deeper penetration for G-Spot stimulation. It will also allow for some clitoral stimulation as he is on top.

1. The female should lie down on her back with her legs raised up and apart. She may use her arms flat on the bed to support her or hold on to both legs until the male is in position.

2. The male should lie down on his stomach and face her, much like the missionary position.

3. Using his arms to support his weight, the male should guide his penis towards the vagina for penetration.

4. The female should keep her legs wide apart during intercourse.

5. Once the male is in position, he can push forward to help keep the female's legs up. She can then use her arms for support by placing them flat on the bed beside her.

Squat

This is a simple and commonly used position. The male should lay on his back on top of a bed. The female should straddle on top and lower herself slowly, guiding the penis into her vagina.

The female is again in control in this position and should raise herself up and down, using the bed or the male's chest to support herself.

There is a reason that this is one of the most used positions – it's great for sensation! And gives the female a good workout. The male also has quite easy access to the clitoris to help stimulation when reaching orgasm.

1. The male should lie on his back at the top of a bed, legs only slightly apart and straight.

2. The female should position herself over his waist and lower herself in a squatting position.

3. Once in position, she should guide the penis inside of her.

4. Once inserted, the female can raise herself up and down at her decided pace.

5. The female should be squatting with her feet on the bed in this position i.e. not on her knees.

One Up

This is an oral sex position. The female should lay on a bed with her rear close to the edge. She should raise one of her legs and hold it in position by wrapping it around her thigh. The male should kneel between her legs and get down on her!

1. The female should lie down on a bed with her bottom very close to the edge.

2. The female should then raise one of her legs into the air and wrap her foot around her other thigh.

3. The male can then kneel on the floor facing towards her. The male should grab hold of the female's body and engage in oral sex.

4. During this position, the female can shift her bodyweight to dictate where the male stimulates her.

This is great foreplay before sex.

Face to Face

In this position, you should sit opposite your partner and the female should slide herself on to the male's lap and sit on top of him. She should wrap her legs around his body until they are touching behind him. The male should then do the same and cradle her bum. Rock back and forth together and get close!

1. Both the male and female should sit opposite each other and face towards one another.

2. The male should cross his legs and allow the female to shift on top and sit on his lap.

3. The female should wrap her legs around the male until her feet are touching behind him. She can then allow for penetration.

4. Once inserted, the male should also wrap his legs around the female and cradle her bum.

5. Both the male and female should now rock back and forth for intimate and close intercourse.

This is a great one for getting intimate – it is a slow pace and is great for stimulation building up to an orgasm. There is also a lot of clitoral stimulation during this one.

The Stand-Up

The female should turn and face a wall several feet away with her bum slightly suck out. The wall should be used as support. The male should then gently insert his penis – he can bend his knees to lower himself if there is difficulty finding access!

1. The female should turn and face a wall several feet away from her.

2. The female should lean forwards and rest her forearms against the wall for support. Her bottom should be slightly tucked out.

3. The female may slightly bend her knees for additional comfort if necessary.

4. The male should approach the female from behind. He should grab hold of her waist and slowly penetrate. The male may also find that he needs to slightly bend his knees before penetrating if there is difficulty getting access from behind.

5. The male can then thrust back and forth. He may hold on to the waist of the female. He may also hold on to her shoulders with his arms straight. If so, the female should slightly arch her back inwards.

The great thing about this is that the female can thrust backwards as the male thrust forwards so you can both control the speed of things!

Hobby Horse

This position requires a chair. Make sure it is reliable and strong.

The male should lay back down on the chair, keeping his body parallel to the ground. The female can then saddle up facing away from him and with her feet on his knees.

1. The male should lie with is back down across the body of a chair. He may use his arms to support him by placing his hand firmly on the floor. His feet should be firmly on the floor.

2. The female should then position herself with her legs either side of the male's waist (facing away from him) and squat to allow penetration.

3. The female should then lean back and rest her hands on either the male's chest area or the chair's edges.

4. Finally, the female should bend her knees and lift her legs so that her feet and resting on the male's knees.

5. The female can then thrust back and forth to engage in intercourse.

6. Once the female is in position, instead of keeping his hands on the floor, the male may grasp the female's waist/ breasts for support and stimulation.

This move requires a lot of core strength from the male to hold the position but is a fun one where the female is in control.

The Elevator – Practice Makes Perfect

This is an oral sex position so is great for foreplay.

The male should be standing and the female kneeling in front. This is a basic oral sex position. Be sure to mix up the speed during oral sex to make the experience better for the male.

1. The male should start by getting into a standing position.

2. The female should then kneel in front of him, facing him.

3. The female can then engage in oral sex.

4. The is a very versatile position and the female is free to alter the speed and sensations she provides the male during oral sex. She may also use her hands while doing so.

5. Alternatively, the male may thrust towards the mouth of the female while she holds her head steady. She may also benefit from the male using his hands to help hold her head in place.

The more you practice, the better you get!

Carpet Burn

In this position, the male should be kneeling on a carpet, bringing one knee in front of him. The female should then kneel in front of him and move to allow him to penetrate her. She should use his body for support and both can begin to thrust.

1. The male should kneel on a carpet with one knee bent out in front of him.

2. The female should kneel in front of the male, facing him. The female should also have one knee bent out in front of her but this must be the opposite knee to the male.

3. The female should then shuffle towards the male and slot herself between his knees; her bent knee outside of his knee, and her knee on the floor inside his bent knee.

4. Once in position, she may allow penetration and both can thrust towards one another.

BEWARE OF CARPET BURN. The name says it all although that's where the excitement comes from!

The Lotus Blossom

The male should go first, sitting with crossed legs. The female straddles on top and wraps her legs around him tightly. She can begin moving once he has penetrated, and he can help by raising her up and down.

1. The male should begin by sitting with his legs crossed.

2. The female should then sit on his lap and allow penetration while facing towards him.

3. The female should then very tightly wrap her legs around the male.

4. Once in position, the male should place his hands underneath the female's bottom and help raise her firmly up and down, pulling her towards him back down

In this position, the male has easy access to the female's upper body so is great for kissing and being intimate. Just make sure you are both comfortable before you begin!

Bridge

The male should lay across two sturdy objects with his body hanging between them. The female should sit on top of him from the side. She should then slowly bring one of her legs up and over so that she is now facing outwards to the side of her partner.

1. The male should lay across two study objects (such as two fixed countertops) and allow his body to hang between them. The male should face upwards towards the ceiling and may require pillows/ blankets for comfort on his shoulders and legs.

2. The female should mount on top of the male with her legs either side of his waist.

3. The female can then allow penetration.

4. The female should slowly raise one of her legs, using the male's body for support, and bring her leg over to the side so that she is now facing sideways from the male. It may help to imagine sitting on a park bench looking outwards.

5. Finally, once in position, the female can begin rocking gently or rotating her hips in a circular motion.

Golden Arch

In this position, have the male sit down with his legs straight, leaning back supporting his weight with his arms out behind him. The female should then sit on top of him and slide herself on to the penis, carefully. She should then bend her knees with her feet situated behind him and begin rocking back and forth.

1. The male should sit down with his legs out straight.

2. The male should lean backwards with his arms out straight behind him for support.

3. The female should then position herself above the male's waist and squat down for penetration. Once penetrated, she should lean back with her arms straight out behind her for support.

4. Finally, the female should position her legs behind the male by bending her knees and placing her feet towards where his hands are situated on the bed.

5. Once in position, the female can begin rocking back and forth.

This is a great position as you can both see each other's bodies and have complete control over the speed and depth of penetration.

Spin Cycle

This is a fun one! The male should sit on top of a washing machine with the setting that makes the most vibration. The female should saddle up on top of him, facing away and help him access the vagina.

1. First, the male should sit on top of a washing machine. The washing machine should have a load on already when trying this position!

2. The female should position herself by standing in front of the male and facing away from him.

3. The female can then begin moving backwards until she can saddle up on top of the male.

4. The female should help guide the penis in for penetration.

5. The male may use one arm behind him on the washing machine for support, and the other can be used to stimulate the clitoris. Alternatively, both arms can be placed behind for support.

This position gives deep penetration with the added benefit of vibrations from the washing machine! This will quickly bring you both to orgasm. If nothing else, the excitement of having sex outside of the bedroom is a great benefit in itself!

Female on Top

The male should lay down on his back with his legs out in front of him. The female should then climb on top and let him penetrate her. She can then lean back to hold on to his ankles or come forward to get close and intimate.

1. The male should lie down on his back with his legs out in front of him.

2. The female should position herself above the male's waist and squat down for penetration. At this point, the female should transition from the squatting position to kneeling with one leg or the male. She should be facing towards him.

3. Once in position, the female is free to come close, sit up or lean back and place her hands on the male's feet for support and control. If she does so, she will easily be able to stimulate her clitoris herself.

This is a good one for the female as she is in control of everything. He can also have a great view of her body during sex.

The Manhandle

For this position, the female should stand in front of the male and face away in a position that provides easy access for penetration. The male should then enter her (this is usually easiest when the female is bent over). She should then slowly straighten up, making sure that the penis remains inside her. When you are both ready and comfortable, start thrusting.

1. The female must start by standing in front of the male but facing away from him.

2. The female should then bend over slightly with her bottom outwards.

3. The male can then approach from behind for penetration, holding on to the female's waist for support.

4. Once inserted, the female should begin slowly standing up straighter.

5. The male can then begin thrusting.

6. The male can have easy access to kiss the female's neck and stimulate both the breasts and the clitoris in this position. The female can also reach behind and grab the male's head to bring it forward for kissing and getting intimate.

The benefit of this position is that it can be done anytime, anywhere! With or without furniture. Inside or out. It is great on if you can reach orgasm through different types of stimulation.

Crossed Keys

The female should lay down with her bum near the edge of the bed. She should cross her legs and raise them into the air. The male should then stand in front and penetrate her. He can then play with her legs during sex, crossing and uncrossing them to change things.

1. The female should sit on the edge of a bed with her feet on the floor.

2. The female should then lean right back until she is laid on the bed.

3. Now, the female can raise her legs and cross them. Her legs should be lifted right up into the air causing a slight elevation of her bottom.

4. The male can now approach from her front for penetration. He should hold the female's legs while doing so.

5. Finally, while having intercourse, the male should play around with her legs, crossing and uncrossing them when he pleases for different sensations.

This position can offer alterations quickly during sex to change the depth of penetration and offer different sensation. This one feels great.

Melody Maker

You will need a chair or something similar to start this position. First, the female should sit on the chair and lean back to point her head downwards. The male should then kneel between her legs and penetrate the vagina. He should hold her hands to offer support if she needs it.

1. The female should sit down on a chair.

2. She should then lean right back until her head is pointing downwards (this might take some core strength!).

3. The male should then kneel and approach her for penetration.

4. Once inserted, it is best to hold on to each other's hand for support and intimacy. This will also maintain stability when things get going.

The idea behind this position is that it increases the blood rush so the female can have an incredible orgasm!

The Peg

The male should begin by laying on his side. His legs should be stretched. The female can then curl on to her side in the opposite direction so that her head is top and tail with his. She should bring her knees up to her chest and put her legs around outside his. He can then penetrate her.

1. The male should lay down on his side on a bed with his legs stretched out straight.

2. She should also lay down on her side in the same position. However, the female's head should be where the male's feet are and she should be facing him.

3. Finally, the female should curl up by bringing her knees up to her chest.

4. From this position, the male should penetrate and slowly begin thrusting.

This does seem confusing, but once you try it, it will make a lot more sense and you will soon be able to get in position in no time!

Galloping Horse

The male should sit on a chair and stretch out his legs. The female should sit on top of him and slide down on to his penis. Her legs should be stretched out behind him. He should hold on to her arms to allow her to lean back. The female can then bring herself forward and back during sex.

1. The male should sit on a sturdy chair with his legs stretched out straight.

2. The female should position herself over the male facing him. She can then lower herself on to his penis for insertion.

3. Once inserted, the male should hold on to the female's hands in a firm grip.

4. Finally, the female should extend her legs out behind the male and the chair. She can then lean right back and begin thrusting back and forth.

5. Ensure that both partners are always holding on to one another's hands as the female is leaning back! She can also use this grip to launch herself forward as she reaches orgasm and wrap her arms around his shoulders for intimacy and support.

This position can offer the male a great view while also giving the female deep penetration. This one is a win/ win position.

Edge of Heaven

The male should begin by sitting on the edge of a bed or a chair. His feet should be down on the floor. The female would then climb on top of his lap with her legs either side of him. You can hold each other's hands for support and stop you from falling backwards.

1. The male should begin by sitting on the edge of a bed or a chair.

2. The male's feet should be down on the floor.

3. The female can now, while facing him, mount herself on the male's lap with her legs flaying out either side of him.

4. Both partners should hold each other's hands for support so that neither fall backwards.

5. Alternatively, the female can hold on to the male's shoulders while he places his hands behind him to support his weight.

In this position, both partners can move as slowly or as quickly as you like. It is a great one for deep penetration and G-spot stimulation. It is also a good one for staying in sync with your partner as you are both supporting each other.

Reverse Spoons

Lay in bed with your partner and both face the same way. He can then spoon her from behind and can begin thrusting. This is a simple position that is good for intimate sex.

1. The female should begin by laying on her side slightly curled up so that she does not lose balance.

2. The male should assume the same position from behind. Both the male and female should be facing the same way.

3. Once in position, the male can penetrate the female from behind. It may be helpful if the female raises her outer leg while he penetrates.

4. Once inserted, the male can begin thrusting. The female can also thrust back towards the male.

Good Spread

The male should lay down on his back. The female should then sit on top of him and slide down on to his penis, slowly starting to spread her legs as wide as she can.

The female is in control in this position – the wider her legs are the deeper the penetration will be.

1. The male should lie down on his back with his legs slightly apart and bent.

2. The female should position herself over the male's waist facing him. She can then squat down to allow for penetration.

3. The female should lean back slightly using her arms for support either on the bed or on the male's legs.

4. Finally, the female should open her legs as wide as possible for deeper penetration and a great view for the male.

The Bullet

The female should lay face up on a bed and have her legs going straight up at a right angle to her body. The partner should kneel behind and start to thrust, using the upright legs as leverage. He can push the legs close together to get a better sensation inside of you, or further apart for deeper penetration.

1. The female should start by lying flat down on a bed facing the ceiling.

2. She should raise her legs to a right angle from her body.

3. The male should then position himself in front of the female on his knees.

4. The male can then shuffle forward for penetration. It may be easier if the female slightly lifts her bottom while this happens.

5. Finally, the male can begin thrusting.

6. While having intercourse, the male can use the female's upwards legs as leverage to get harder thrusts. He can also close her legs together while they are in the air to get a better sensation himself.

A general rule of thumb – the wider the legs, the deeper the penetration; the tighter the legs, the better the sensation for the male!

Kneeling Dog

The female should get down on her hands and knees and lean forward on to her arms. The male can get behind in the doggy position and the female can sit back on to his lap.

1. The female should begin by getting down on her hands and knees on a bed or the floor.

2. She should then lower her arms so that she is bent down closer to the floor. Her bottom should remain in the same position up in the air.

3. The female should slightly arch her back inwards ensuring that her bottom remains up.

4. The male can now kneel behind her and approach her for penetration.

5. Once inserted, the female can slowly lift her body back up until she is kneeling on his lap and begin thrusting back and forth. The male has very good access for breast and clitoral stimulation in this position.

Alternatively, the female can remain with her body close to the floor and thrust in an upwards and downwards motion. It's best to mix up to two different variations during sex!

This is a great one for the male and will get him going! It also allows for great penetration and friction with the vagina so is one of the best! You might want to write this one down...

Back Breaker

The female should lay on a bed with her legs off the edge as well as her bum. The male should kneel and penetrate. The female can then arch her back. The male can then thrust.

1. The female should start by sitting on the edge of a bed.

2. Next, she needs to lie right back so that her head is on the bed. A pillow should be placed under her back to create an arch.

3. The female should now shuffle forward slightly so that her bottom is now off the edge of the bed.

4. The male should now kneel on the floor facing her. He can now grab hold of the female's bottom and penetrate.

5. The male can now thrust and should keep his hands on the female's bottom.

In this position, the male can hold on to the female's bum while having sex or a pillow can be used to support underneath it. The arch in the female's back is key to enhancing the orgasm – it can be very easy to hit the G-spot by only making small changes in the back's position.

Pretzel Dip

The female should lay on her side and have her partner straddle the leg on the bed. The other leg should wrap around his waist.

1. The female should begin by lying down on her side on a bed.

2. The female should raise her outer leg into the air while the male gets into position.

3. The male should kneel over the female's leg (the leg which is still on the bed).

4. The male should then shuffle forward until close to the female's waist.

5. The female should then wrap her leg (the leg in the air) around the front of the male's waist.

6. The male should then grab the leg and lift it until he can penetrate.

7. The male should keep hold of this leg as he begins thrusting.

G-Spot

The female should begin by lying on her stomach and then transitioning to face sideways in one direction. She can then bend her legs at the knee to support herself and keep balance. The male should approach her from behind on his knees for penetration. Once inserted, he may hold on to her waist while thrusting for harder and faster sex.

1. The female should start getting into a sideways position. She can bend her legs for support and balance.

2. Once in position, the male should kneel behind her and approach for penetration. It may help if the female opens her legs slightly for easier access.

3. Once inserted, the female can close her legs and the male can hold on to her hips while he thrusts.

This one is designed to hit the G-spot! So, keep that in mind! The male does all of the work in this position and it is designed for stimulating the female orgasm so enjoy!

This is also a great position when you want to start with one thing and end with another. For example, it's very easy to transition from this position to missionary or even doggy style during sex.

Slippery Nipple

The male should sit upright as the female lies flat on her back. She should place her legs either side of the male and inch forward. He can then do all the work during sex. The female can lie back and enjoy.

1. The female should begin by lying down on her back facing the ceiling.

2. The female should spread her legs wide and bend them at the knee with her feet flat.

3. The male should kneel in front.

4. The female should inch forward towards the male until he can penetrate her.

5. Once inserted, the male has full control to lean back, but can lean right forward into a lowered missionary position and stimulate the nipples with his mouth.

The Clasp

The male should begin by standing up. The female can wrap herself around his waist and he can hold her up by placing his hands on her back and bum. Allow careful penetration and the female can raise herself up and down while the male carries her.

1. This is a standing position and requires upper body strength. The male should begin by standing up. It may help for him to stand against a wall, to begin with.

2. The female should approach him facing towards him.

3. The female should wrap her arms around the male's shoulders and he should grab hold of her behind her back and under her bottom.

4. Simultaneously, the female should lift off the ground and the male should help lift her up and above his waist.

5. The male should then carefully lower the female to his penis for penetration ensuring that he is still supporting her back and bottom.

6. Once inserted, both the male and female should help intercourse by supporting the female moving in an up and downward thrust.

If you are struggling with this position, it can be done against a wall rather than away from it. This way, the wall can support a significant portion of the female's weight and firmer thrusts can take place.

This is another position which can be done anywhere. It may require some upper body strength from the male – it can be quite hard to hold someone up for very long! It may be helpful if the female leans back against a wall or something else to support her during sex.

Reverse Cowgirl

This is a popular classic. The male should lay down flat on his back and the female should straddle on top of him, facing away instead of towards his face. The female can then move back and forth in complete control of the pace of sex.

1. The male should lie down on a bed facing upwards. His legs should be slightly bent and slightly apart.

2. The female should position herself over the male's waist and face away from him towards his feet.

3. The female can kneel with one leg on either side of the male's waist. She can then allow for penetration.

4. Once inserted, the female can begin thrusting back and forth.

The control from this is a great one for women and is often a popular position – some women find that they can't finish until they are on top and in control. The male benefits from having to do little work and gets a great view from behind. This can be quite a turn on.

Tight Squeeze

This is a position for adventurous sex and is best done somewhere other than the bedroom.

The female should sit down somewhere and wrap her legs around her partner and 'tight squeeze'. The male should be standing, and the female's arms can wrap around him for support. This allows for close and intimate sex wherever you are.

1. The female should find somewhere sturdy and secure to sit up on to such as a kitchen countertop or a table.

2. The female should then shuffle close to the edge and open her legs. She may find it useful to position her hands behind her for support at this stage.

3. The male can then approach from the front and position himself between her legs for penetration.

4. Once inserted, the female should wrap her legs tightly around the male's body and squeeze, bringing him close.

5. The female can now finally also wrap her arms around the male's neck and shoulders.

6. Finally, although the male is in control during intercourse, the female is in a great position to influence the male's thrusts and movements.

Lust and Thrust

The female should lay down on her back off the edge of the bed with her feet on the floor. She should raise her body and support herself on her arms with elbows bent. The partner should stand in front for penetration and lean down with his arms on either side of her body.

1. The female should lie down on her back on a bed with her bottom and legs off the edge of the bed.

2. The female should raise her body from the bottom down by positioning her elbows on the bed to support her and use her arms to lift.

3. The male should now position himself in front of the female and penetrate the female.

4. Finally, the male should lean forward and position his arms either side of the female's body during intercourse.

5. Alternatively, the male may remain standing and hold on to the female's waist while thrusting.

This position is great for getting close and intimate during sex without compromising thrust or pace. There is minimal work for the female to do during this position and both partners are well supported and secured.

Afternoon Delight

The female should lay on her side and slightly raise her outer leg to allow easier access. The male should penetrate from the side. Once inserted, the female can relax and lower her outer leg back down to the resting position.

1. The female should begin by lying down on her side. She should maintain a slight bend in her legs at the knee.

2. The female should slightly raise her outer leg to allow easier access for penetration. It may be useful for the female to use her hands to help support her leg while in the air.

3. The male should approach from behind the female and shuffle into position for penetration.

4. Once inserted, the female can relax her outer leg and lower is back to the resting position.

5. The male is then free to thrust gently.

This is a good lazy position when you want to have sex, but don't have much energy!

Half on, Half off

The female should start by laying on a bed, legs off the end. The male can then stand and penetrate while the female wraps her legs around his.

1. The female should begin by lying down on the edge of the bed. Her legs should be hanging off the edge.

2. The female should open her legs outwards to allow access for the male.

3. The male can now approach from the front and position himself for penetration.

4. Once inserted, the female should lift her legs and wrap them around the males before having sex. If the bed is low, the male can kneel instead.

This is a good one for reaching the G-spot without having to do too much work!

The Ship

The male should lay down on his back. The female should then sit down on his penis and face sideways so that both legs are over on one side of his body.

1. The male should begin by lying down in the basic position on a bed i.e. facing upwards, legs slightly bent and apart.

2. The female should now position herself above the waist. However, she should face to the side of the male and both feet should be next to each other on only one side of the male.

3. The female can down lower herself to allow for penetration.

4. Both of the female's legs should now be on one side of the male's body. The female may now position her hands behind her on the opposite side of the male's body.

This is a position where the female is in control and can be good if she needs to be on top to finish.

The female should begin by lying face down on the bed. She should move closer to the edge so that her head and upper body hang off the bed towards to floor, using her hands for support. The male can then penetrate.

1. The female should begin by lying face down on a bed.

2. The female should now shuffle towards the edge of the bed and position herself so that her head and upper body completely hang off the edge. She may need to use her hands and arms to support her weight on the floor.

3. The male should kneel now behind the female to penetrate from behind. This is best done from a kneeling position behind her with legs either side of the female.

4. The male can now penetrate.

5. The male should help support the female's body while she is hanging off the bed. This can be done by firmly holding on to the female's waist, or by having the male hold on to the female's hands and pulling them back. This is best for when things get rough!

Again, this position is designed for the ultimate orgasm with an increased blood flow to the head and all the effort being done by the male.

The Cat

The male lies down on top of the female in the missionary position. He then penetrates her as much as he can, bringing his body up against hers. Instead of thrusting, he can then move his hips in small circles to stimulate the clitoris with the bottom of his penis.

1. The female should begin by lying down face up on a bed with her legs slightly bent and apart.

2. The male should now position himself on top in the missionary position.

3. The male can now penetrate.

4. Once inserted, the male can push upwards into the female's body so that he is positioned slightly further to cause more stimulation on the clitoris.

5. Finally, instead of thrusting, the male should rotate his hips in a circular motion to cause more friction on the clitoris and increase stimulation.

This is great for women who need clitoral stimulation to orgasm. Just make sure both of you are comfortable in the position. It is very easy to switch between the standard missionary position and this position, so try mixing it up!

Closed for Business

This is an oral sex position. The female should lay down on her back with her legs 'closed for business'. The male can then go down on her.

1. The female should lie down on her back and face upwards. Her legs should remain closed and together, but completely straight.

2. Secondly, the female should raise her hips into the air and position her feet behind her head as shown in the illustration.

3. The male can now kneel over her legs, facing her.

4. The male can now lean forward and begin having oral sex with the female.

This position emphasises clitoral stimulation.

Happy Birthday!

The male should lie down on a bed with his feet on the floor. The female should get on top with her legs and guide his penis into her vagina.

1. The male should lie down on a bed but ensure that his feet remain on the floor.

2. The female should now position herself over the male's waist a face him.

3. The female can now lower herself down to allow for penetration. Once inserted, the female should assume a kneeling position with one leg or the male's.

4. The female can now begin thrusting back and forth or, if she leans forward towards the male's chest, she can thrust up and down.

The best part about this is that the female is in overall control, but the male can use his legs to help thrust and get faster when reaching climax. He also gets a great view.

Organ Grinder

The female should lie on her back with her legs apart and raise them into the air. The partner should kneel down and forward between her legs. He can then hold the legs up as he thrusts.

1. The female should lie on her back with her legs apart and bent. The female should raise her legs into the air. She may find it helpful to use her hands to support her legs up in this position until the male is in position.

2. The male can now kneel in front of the female and move forward between her legs.

3. The male can now penetrate the female.

4. Once inserted, the male should hold on to the female's legs and keep them up in the air while he thrusts. By holding the female's thighs, the male can use her legs to help him provide firmer thrusts.

This is a great one for reaching the G-spot and finishing sex.

The Mermaid

Find a flat surface and have the female lay down facing up with her bum at the edge. A pillow or something similar should be used to raise the hips safely and comfortably. The female should raise her legs above and keep them closed. The male can then stand and penetrate – he can hold on to her legs to keep them secured.

1. The female should find a flat surface such as a bed, kitchen countertop or table. A pillow can be used for comfort and support.

2. The female should raise her legs right up into the air as a 90-degree angle to her body. She should keep them closed and keep her feet together. She may use her hand to support her legs in this position until the male is in position.

3. The male can now approach from the front in a standing position and penetrate the female.

4. The male should hold on to the legs and keep them in the air and together.

5. The female can now place her hands by her side for support. Alternatively, she can place her elbows behind her and support herself from this position.

Again, keeping the legs together will cause a greater sensation for the male where there is more rubbing on the inside of the vagina. The elevation is used to make it easier to hit the G-spot.

Pretzel

The female should lay on her side, have her partner straddle her leg and bring the other leg around his waist. This gives good penetration and the male will have his hands free for clitoral stimulation or support if needed.

1. The female should lie down on her side. Her legs should be straight at this point.

2. The male should kneel over the lower leg and lift the female's outer leg while he approaches for penetration.

3. This leg outer leg should now be wrapped around the front of the male's waist.

4. The male can now penetrate.

5. Once inserted, the male may use his hands for support or he may stimulate the clitoris.

Back Breaker

The female should lie on the bed with her legs hanging off the edge. She should shift her bum forward until it is also just off the edge. The male should kneel in front of her and penetrate. The female can push up with her toes and arch her back. The male can then hold up her bum and thrust.

1. The female should begin by lying down on a bed with her legs off the edge and her feet. She should be facing upwards.

2. The male should approach from the front for penetration.

3. Once inserted, the female should use her feet to push her body upwards and cause an arch in her back.

4. When arched, the male should grab hold of the females bottom to help her maintain the position and begin thrusting.

This position requires most effort to be done by the male, but having the female push with her toes and change the arch in her back can make it much easier to hit the G-spot.

The Bumper Car

This is a thrilling sex position which allows for deep penetration. This is great if you require G-spot stimulation to reach orgasm. Again, this position requires penile flexibility, so make sure the male is comfortable with the position.

Start with the female laying down on her stomach with her legs wide open and straight out. The male should then lie down on his stomach, with his legs open and straight out. He must be facing in the opposite direction. Afterwards, the male reverses back towards his partner so his thighs are resting over hers. He needs to do this until he can point his penis towards his partner's vagina. Then penetrate slowly.

1. The female should lie down on her stomach facing downwards. Her legs should be open as wide as comfortably possible and straight.

2. The male should position himself facing away from the female by her feet.

3. The male should also lie down on his stomach, legs open wide and straight.

4. Once in position, the male should slowly begin moving backwards so that his thighs rest over the female's.

5. From this point, the male should focus on guiding his penis towards the vagina and penetrate slowly, ensuring that both partners are comfortable.

6. Once inserted, the male can begin thrusting back and forth.

Safety Tips

This position requires penile flexibility. If you want to find out if the male's penis is flexible enough, have him stand against a wall. Pull his penis gradually down. If the penis can point directly down to the ground without causing pain then you should be fine to perform this position, but still be careful. The female should stay still when the male is initially penetrating her. The female should wait while he finds the most comfortable position and angle to thrust without injury.

Butter Churner

For this position, the female should lay on her back and bring her feet over her head so that the bum is up in the air. The male should stand over and squat up and down, coming completely out of the vagina.

1. The female should lie down on her back.

2. The female should bring her legs right up so that her bottom is in the air and bring her feet back over her head.

3. The male should now stand in front of the female with his feet by her bottom.

4. The male should now squat down for penetration.

5. Once inserted, the male should continue squatting up and down, penetrating and re-penetrating the female.

This position will feel like the male is penetrating for the first time every time he penetrates which can be satisfying.

Kneel and Sit

The male should kneel on a bed and the female should straddle him with her legs either side. The female has to control and choice in this position – sit, grind or move up and down. It's up to you!

1. The male should begin by kneeling on a bed or anywhere else that seems comfortable.

2. The female should approach the male from the front and straddle his lap with one leg on either side of the male. The female should be on her feet rather than on her knees and be facing away from the male.

3. The female can then position herself to allow for penetration.

The male has good access to the female's upper body in this position.

Wraparound

The male should sit on a floor with his legs out. The female should straddle and wrap her legs around him and carefully allow him to penetrate her.

1. The male should sit down on the floor with his legs out in front of him.

2. The female should position herself above the male, facing him and with one foot either side of the male's legs.

3. The female can now lower herself to allow for penetration.

4. Once inserted, the female should wrap her legs around the back of the male.

5. For support, the male can either wrap his arms around the female or lean back on his arms.

This position is great as it gives some control back to the male. You can stay close and kiss while having sex without compromising the amount of penetration.

The Landslide

The female should begin by laying down looking at the floor. She should rest upon her forearms with her legs apart. The partner should sit behind and over her legs, also leaning back on his arms behind him. He should then penetrate and begin having sex.

1. The female should start by lying face down on the floor.

2. The female places her forearms below her chest and rest on them. Her legs should also be apart at this point.

3. The male should then sit behind the female on his knees. His legs should be over hers and on both sides i.e. outside of her legs.

4. The male can now position himself to allow for penetration.

5. Once inserted, the male should lean back on his hands with his arms stretched out behind him.

By having the female close her legs, the male will feel fuller inside and it is much easier to find the G-spot.

Lap

This is a simple position. The male should sit up, using a wall or headboard to support him. The female sits on top and both can rock together.

1. The male should sit up in front of a wall or a headboard with his legs crossed.

2. The female can now position herself facing towards the male and above his lap.

3. The female should now lower herself in a squat to allow for penetration. She can remain with her feet on the floor or her knees.

4. Once inserted, the female is in control and can rock back and forth.

This is a good position for a long sex session.

Home Fitness

In this position, both the male and female get into the push-up position. The female should be on the bottom and can use her knees to support. The male penetrates her from behind. This is a VERY exhausting position but can be worth the effort!

1. The female should begin by getting into a press-up position. She may find it easier to rest on her knees.

2. The male should position himself over the female in the press-up position.

3. The male should carefully penetrate the female – he may use one of his arms to help penetrate if he has the strength to hold up his weight on one arm.

Shoulder Stand

The female should start by being on her back and the male should kneel in front. She should wrap her legs around and allow him to penetrate. He supports her with one hand on her back and she can then shift all her weight onto her shoulders. He can now thrust.

1. The female should begin by lying down on her back with her legs open and slightly bent.

2. The male should kneel in front of the female and move towards her to allow for penetration.

3. Once inserted, the female should wrap her legs tightly around the male's back and bottom.

4. The male should now place either one or both hands on the female's back to support her.

5. The female can now lift her back until her shoulders support all of her weight. She should maintain this arch position throughout intercourse.

The be secure and safe, the male should always provide support to the female.

This position allows for very deep penetration and incredible orgasms.

Dinner Time

The female should sit on a sofa on the edge. The partner should kneel in front and be between her legs. He can hold her thighs to get some more control as he engages in oral sex.

1. The female should sit straight up on the edge of a sofa. Alternatively, she can lean back flat.

2. The male should kneel in front of the female and take hold of her thighs.

3. he male should spread the female's legs wide and engage in oral sex.

4. The female should relax her legs so that the male has full control of their position throughout oral sex. If she resists or has impulses, the male should restrain her from moving – he is in control!

Face Sitter

This is an oral sex position – the name says it all here!

The male should lay down on his back. The female should lower herself above his face. Do NOT put all your weight down – the female should support herself using a wall or the bed. The female is in complete control of where his tongue is going.

1. The male should lack down on his back.

2. The female should position herself over the male's head facing either way.

3. The female can now squat down until the male can begin oral sex.

4. The female must remember to support all of her weight throughout this position. She is in total control of how the male's mouth is positioned and what it does.

The Thigh Master

This position is a variation of the cowgirl position. To begin with, the female should be on top facing away from the male. The male's knees should be raised to give the female something to support her.

1. The male should lie down in his back with his legs apart and slightly bent.

2. The female should position herself above his waist and face towards him.

3. The female can now kneel with one leg either side of the male to allow for penetration.

4. Once inserted, the male should bend his legs further while keeping his feet firmly flat.

5. The female should rest back against the male's bent legs as she uses her hips only to thrust back and forth.

Being on top is generally great for the female orgasm, but having the male's knees up will make his sensation better inside the female and you can both have a better orgasm together.

The Staircase

The female should sit on some stairs with her back leaning against one of the walls. The male should be standing a bit further down. The female should lift one leg up as the male penetrates her. He can then begin thrusting.

Just make sure no one else is around!

1. Locate an appropriate staircase!

2. Have the female sit on the staircase several steps up from the male. This will depend on both partners' height so you may need to find what is most comfortable for you both.

3. The female should lift one of her legs onto the male's shoulders and rest there throughout this position.

4. The male can then penetrate, use the female's raised leg for support, and aid with firmer thrusts.

Kneeling Wheelbarrow

This one is easier than the one we tried earlier! The female starts on all fours, putting her weight on to one forearm and one knee. The partner then kneels behind and penetrates the vagina. This is another great one for hitting to G-spot.

1. The female should start by getting down on her hands and knees.

2. The female should then move on to her forearms instead of on her hands.

3. The female should now rest all of her weight on one of her forearms and one of her knees on the same side.

4. The male should now kneel behind the female and penetrate, holding on to both of the female's upper legs when thrusting.

Dinner is Served

The female should wrap her legs around her partner and hold her bum in a carrying position. He should then penetrate. The female can then begin to lean back until parallel to the floor.

1. The male should begin by standing in front of the female.

2. The female should then hold on to the male's shoulders, jump up and wrap her legs around the back of the male. Think of this as a carrying position.

3. The female should then allow for penetration.

4. Once inserted, the male should grab a firm hold of the female's hands and lean right back until her body is parallel.

5. The female can now begin using her legs to help her thrust up and down.

This position is really fun and for both partners. It does require some upper body strength though! If this position is too difficult in terms of strength required, the female can rest her back on a bed instead of being elevated in the air parallel to the ground.

Ballet

This is an exhaustive position that requires flexibility, stamina and strength from both partners. Rather than a unique sex position, this is better thought of as an exciting way to begin having sex.

The female must begin by standing on a surface close to other structures that can be used for support such as a wall or cabinet. She should then lunge forward and lower herself, while the male does the same. He should inch closer to penetrate. Either party can now control the depth of penetration for the best orgasm.

1. The female should begin by standing on a surface close to other firm surroundings such as walls or heavy/ fitted furniture.

2. The male should be standing in front of her.

3. Once in position, the male should ready himself to catch the female and support her body weight.

4. The female should lunge forward towards the male. He should be ready to support her. The male should catch the female by holding her under the shoulders. When caught, she should be positioned around the male's shoulder area.

5. The male can then lower the female while she keeps her legs out straight to the sides.

6. Penetration can then take place.

Balance is key! Be sure to use surrounding supports in case!

Leg Up!

You should both begin by facing each other. The female should raise one leg and wrap it around the male's leg, pulling him closer.

1. Both the male and female should begin by standing and facing one another.

2. The female should raise one leg and bend it at the knee.

3. The female should then use her leg and wrap it around the male's. She can then use her leg to bring him closer for penetration to take place.

4. The female should keep her leg wrapped around the male for the entirety of this position.

This is great when you can't find a bedroom to have sex or just want to mix things up a bit!

Dirty Dancing

This is another anywhere, anytime move but the support of a sturdy object may be helpful when you haven't tried it before.

The male should lean on a wall facing the female and hold her. She should straddle him and wrap her legs around for balance.

1. The male should lean back against a wall, facing the female.

2. The female should hop up on to the male and wrap her legs around his back. He should use his hands to support her from the bottom.

3. The female should now allow for penetration.

4. Once inserted, the female can use the male's shoulders to help her move up and down during sex.

This is an intimate position where the male has a lot of access to the female's upper body. The penetration and clitoral stimulation can be controlled easily.

Leapfrog

Leapfrog is very much like the doggy style that was covered earlier in this book – it is a variation of the doggy position.

You should start in the typical doggy style pose, but the female should lower her head and arms so that they are resting on the bed. The partner should then continue to penetrate from behind like usual.

1. The female should begin by getting down on her hands and knees facing away from the male.

2. The female should lower her upper body by transitioning from resting on her hands to resting on her forearms. Her bottom should remain up in the air and she should arch her back inwards.

3. The male should kneel behind the female, just like the doggy style, and approach for penetration.

4. The male can then thrust firmly.

The great thing about this position is that penetration becomes much deeper than usual and frees up the hands. It is also great for getting a bit rougher than the normal doggy style positions.

69

This is perhaps one of the wider known and popular foreplay positions. For this, the male should lay down facing upwards. The female should straddle on top facing the male's feet end. She should stretch out on top of the male and begin oral sex, while he does the same.

1. The male should begin by lying down on his back on a bed and face upwards. His legs should be slightly apart, but straight.

2. The female should then position herself by kneeling over the male's stomach with one leg either side. She should be facing away towards the male's feet.

3. The female can then begin shuffling backwards until her waist is position above the male's face for oral sex.

4. The male can then engage in oral sex.

5. The female can now lean forward so that her face is above the male's waist. She can then also engage in oral sex at the same time as the male.

Both partners benefit from this position and can be great for stimulation before having sex.

The Hinge

The male should begin by kneeling upon a bed and leaning back to support his weight. The female should face away, positioned in the doggy pose. She should lean down on to her forearms and move backwards until he has penetrated and begin having sex. This is good for keeping control of the penetration and speed.

1. The male should begin by kneeling on a bed and leaning backwards. He should position his arms behind him to help support his weight in this position.

2. The female should then face away from the male in front of him. She should get into the doggy style position i.e. on her hand and knees.

3. The female should lean forward on to her forearms and raise her bottom.

4. The female can now shuffle back towards the male to allow for penetration.

5. Both the male and female can thrust up and down in this position.

The Missionary 180

This position puts a spin on the traditional missionary position, but it requires the male to be flexible!

First, the female needs to lay down on her back with her legs spread apart. The male then lies on top, but with his head down towards her feet – his legs should be on either side of her body. Once in position, the male should carefully push his penis downwards and penetrate his partner. Get comfortable and perform upward and downward thrusts.

1. The female should lie down on her back facing upwards.

2. The male should then position himself on top of the female, but with his head towards her feet. The male should be using his arms to bear weight at this point or be resting his weight on his elbows.

3. The male must now position his legs either side of the female if not done so already.

4. The male should now slowly lower his middle section and begin pushing his penis back and towards the vagina. The female may help guide the penis while the male supports his weight.

5. Once inserted, the male can begin upward and downward thrusts.

Safety Tips

This position requires the male to have a very flexible penis – make sure he is comfortable before committing to the position! There is a risk of him straining his penis's suspensory ligaments. If he does feel any significant pain you should consider leaving the position behind and finding something better suited and comfortable. When entering the position, the female should be careful not to pull hard on the penis while guiding it inside her.

Fourth Book: 74 ILLUSTRATED SEX POSITIONS FOR COUPLES

WHAT'S THE IMPORTANT OF SEX IN YOUR RELATIONSHIP

Beside proliferation, sex is necessary for some reasons in any committed relationship. It is at last about the closeness, joy, and the sexual articulation. Intercourse has numerous definite scholarly, enthusiastic, physical and social advantages. Understanding the advantages will assist couples with perceiving that sex in their connections won't just assistance themselves however help bond their relationship further and make a more extensive feeling of closeness in a caring relationship. Regardless of whether this is a long haul relationship or one that is merely beginning, sex is something imperative to consider for your general wellbeing.

A genuinely dynamic sex life may yield numerous advantages, including an energetic appearance because of better dietary propensities and constant exercise. Studies show that sexual action consumes calories and fat, however can likewise make individuals live increasingly sound lifestyles. Individuals who have sex usually were found to have more significant levels of a neutralizer considered immunoglobulin An (IgA), which, as indicated by specialists at Wilkes University in Pennsylvania, battle sickness and guard the body from colds and this season's flu virus. Sex causes us rest all the more serenely, and through better rest, sex makes a more grounded insusceptible framework. Oxytocin discharged during climax advances a night of increasingly peaceful rest for the two people. Oxytocin helps different zones of the body too. It builds levels of oxytocin to the cerebrum and diminishes heart issues in the two ladies and men. It can help with torment control, as per an investigation led at the Headache Clinic at Southern Illinois University. The examination found that half of the female headache sufferers announced help after peaking. Numerous different sorts of torment have been appeared to diminish when you are sexually dynamic also.

For a lady, there is numerous advantages to having constant sex, for example, encountering lighter periods with less issues. When the uterus contracts it frees the assemblage of issue causing mixes and can remove blood and tissue all the more rapidly, assisting with closure your period quicker. Sex will likewise bring down pulse and increment bladder control, which is significant for ladies after conceiving an offspring. Climax is connected to a decline in prostate malignant growth for men and security against endometriosis for ladies.

Sex is useful for the person's enthusiastic wellbeing, yet additionally for the general strength of the relationship. Sexual fulfillment is firmly connected with the general personal satisfaction. The expansion of sex raises your feeling of prosperity and fulfillment with yourself. Laura Berman, Ph.D., an aide clinical educator of OB-GYN, and Psychiatry at the Feinberg School of Medicine at Northwestern University, says climaxes can diminish worry because of the endorphins that are discharged; these hormones initiate delight focuses in the cerebrum that make sentiments of closeness and unwinding and fight off sadness.

So if you end up lacking sexual want, you might be encountering a hormone lopsidedness. BHRC clinical spa is the pioneer in bio-indistinguishable hormone substitution treatment - a more secure method with better outcomes

When sex is incredible with you and your accomplice in bed, your certainty will increment in different zones. As indicated by sex specialist Sandor Gardos, "When things work out in a good way in bed, you feel progressively certain and incredible in different pieces of your life," along these lines making us all the more brave and uninhibited in life. It helps our confidence, our feeling of being alluring, attractive, capable and sure. Which this way carries constructive reasoning and activities to our own lives. For our connections, our expanded closeness because of adoring physical contact brings about a high measure of oxytocin, discharged during sex and kissing. We built up the inclination to bond, which is the place the longing to snuggle and hold each other originates from. Sex with somebody you are not in adoration with can in any case be pleasurable however doesn't satisfy the enthusiastic need, which is the reason it is smarter to spare this for somebody you care about.

In the wake of conversing with a few wedded couples that have been hitched for a long time or more, I got understanding into how significant sex is in keeping up a stable relationship. All the married couples focused on that sex is significant in a serious relationship because it keeps up a degree of closeness that the two individuals need to succeed. They likewise proposed that it causes one accomplice bond with the other accomplice and makes a feeling of bliss. All concur that it keeps up that supposed "sparkle" that is often required so prop want up all through the riotous life that most couples have with money related duties, social commitment, and youngster raising. Else, it can often feel like you are in a flat mate type association rather than a marriage. Sex between accomplices assists with keeping up a general feeling of prosperity.

Accept a glance at any sex exhortation section on the web, and you'll likely locate a couple of inquiries that start this way: "I'm dating the ideal individual. They're sweet, hot, and amusing. There's only a specific something... " And whether that one thing is a lower (or higher) sex drive, a wrinkle one individual doesn't share, or only an absence of sexual science, the author needs to realize how to make it work. All things considered, how significant is sex in a relationship, truly?

The appropriate response indeed relies upon the unique individuals and relationship, says Megan Fleming, PhD, a couples instructor and sex specialist who rehearses in New York. A few people place a ton of significance on sex, while for other people, it is anything but a need. A couple could engage in sexual relations once in a while or never, yet if the two individuals are content with that, then it is anything but an issue. Be that as it may, others place a great deal of significance on sex, and sexual contradiction can put strain on the relationship.

"When sex is working out in a good way seeing someone's, typically a little piece of a relationship. Be that as it may, when it's not working out positively, tragically, it can cast a shadow on the relationship all in all," Dr. Fleming clarifies.

One regular region of contention is differences in drive, when one accomplice needs to engage in sexual relations more often than the other. "Confidence issues can come up around that," Dr. Fleming says. Right now, says that couples should cooperate to locate a "sweet spot" where they're engaging in sexual relations often enough that they feel associated with one another. One approach to do this is to take into consideration "responsive want" — implying that even though the collaborate with the lower sex drive probably won't feel up for sex at the time, however if the band together with the higher sex drive starts via stroking and contacting them, they may prepare turned on and feel for sex. "That is a decent way individuals can come to and approach sex," Dr. Fleming says. "In any case, if it's more in the feeling of 'take one for the group,' or driving yourself to accomplish something that doesn't feel directly for your body, that generally will be upsetting" for the two individuals, she says.

Another typical territory of contention is sexual brokenness, she says. This incorporates erectile brokenness, difficulty arriving at climax, or conditions that cause torment during intercourse. Contingent upon the individual and the sort of sexual brokenness, there might be masturbation activities or medicines that can help — and the couple can likewise reevaluate how they approach sex to concentrate more on joy than entrance or climax.

Regardless of whether it's a difference in moxie, sexual brokenness, or another zone of contention — one individual has a crimp the other doesn't share; one individual needs to have a go at something that the other individual doesn't; one individual needs an open relationship and the other doesn't — the most ideal approach to move toward this contention is to discuss it with your accomplice (particularly with the assistance of a specialist). Now and again you'll understand you should separate — yet different occasions, you might have the option to cooperate to discover a spot where you're both upbeat.

When discussing sex, Dr. Fleming says it's imperative to utilize positive language. "So often, we talk from dissatisfaction or disillusionment, with you never... " she clarifies. "When you bring it up, you would prefer not to bring it up from dissatisfaction, yet as a matter of fact and the aching. It is anything but a you're not doing it right circumstance, it's encouraging feedback: I truly like it when, it feels great to me, I truly acknowledge, I need to encounter this with you.'"

Another approach to move toward struggle around sex, particularly when it comes to taking a stab at something new, is to try things out by talking about the subject such that is not all that individual — for instance, raising an article or TV appear. You could start by saying something like, "I went over a tenderfoot's manual for hitting today," or "Did you see that open sex on the Ferris wheel scene in Insecure?"

"A great deal of times, the language I advise my customers to utilize is 'I'm befuddled' or 'I'm interested,' because as a rule that gets a non-guarded reaction," Dr. Fleming says. "It's human instinct to need to disclose things to individuals, and interest for the most part draws out a similar vitality in your accomplice."

SECRETS TO KEEPING THE DESIRE ALIVE

Esther clarifies that it's tied in with going to a concession to genuine essential human needs. The principal set being security, wellbeing, dependability, and lastingness. These are tying down and establishing sentiments that we call home. The second being experience, hazard, and the unforeseen. Joining these two extremely differentiating and often clashing arrangements of human needs in a single marriage can be dubious!

A significant test in present day connections is that we anticipate that our accomplice should be everything: our closest companion, our partner, our sweetheart, etc. Esther comments, "We ask what once, a whole town used to give. Having a place, personality, greatness and secret across the board. Give me consistency, yet give me shock."

In her examination, Esther asked individuals when they got themselves generally attracted to their accomplice. Across most societies, sexual orientations, and religions, probably the most widely recognized answers were when they're separated and when they rejoin.

The following arrangement of typical answers were when they saw their accomplice accomplishing something they're energetic about, totally encompassed in, and when they're brilliant and sure. These answers show that individuals are keen on encountering a feeling of secret and slipperiness about their accomplice, yet additionally keeping them close enough.

For the third arrangement of answers, a more significant part of individuals said they were generally attracted to their accomplice when they encountered chuckling, shock, and curiosity.

There's no poverty in want.

So I don't get desire's meaning? As per Esther, "is most intriguing that there's no poverty with regards to want. There is no consideration taking. Care-taking is an enemy of sexual enhancer. Requiring somebody is a shutdown. Anything that raises parenthood diminishes sensual charge."

She clarifies that, "In the oddity among affection and want, the most confusing thing is, that the very fixings that sustain love - correspondence, assurance, are once in a while the very fixings that stifle want."

To continue want, there should be an equalization of necessities.

Esther closes the discussion by sharing that if we need to continue want, there should be an equalization and a compromise of necessities. This incorporates space for sexual protection, foreplay, making a sensual space, and a mindfulness that energy is discontinuous. Couples who see long haul want realize how to carry it back with the component of shock and immediacy.

Sex doesn't need to get exhausting in a long haul marriage. As the years pass by and you get more established, your connection ought to show signs of improvement. Sex with your accomplice can turn out to be all the more fulfilling because you know each other's preferences, aversions, propensities, and inclinations.

We realize that life can disrupt the general flow. Errands, children, accounts, and different issues can discourage sentiment. These ordinary variables can meddle with both your longing for sex and finding an opportunity to invest the exertion. Yet, don't place sex last on the daily schedule. There are approaches to organize sex and keep it energizing.

What You Need for a Healthy Sex Life

Building and keeping up a decent sex life with your accomplice requires both of you to invest energy and exertion. These are the fixings that can assist you with keeping your close connection fulfilling:

Gainful and important communication

Love for one another

Physical fascination

Ability to set aside a few minutes for one another

Date evenings, fun, and liveliness

Acknowledgment of one another's blemishes and idiosyncrasies

There is no motivation behind why you can't have a functioning and stable sex life for some, numerous years. Attempt the methodologies recorded underneath to keep these critical fixings in your marriage.

Keep Your Sex Life Healthy and Strong

There are different approaches to keep things fun and energizing in the room. Attempt any of these strategies to keep sex with your companion fulfilling for both of you.

Great Communication

Correspondence is the way in to a stable and dynamic sex life in a marital relationship, so talk with each other more! Talking about shallow things can be fun, yet make sure to go further to build up closeness truly. Offer your most in-depth considerations and emotions with each other regularly. Sexual closeness is a proceeding with procedure of discovery. Real closeness through correspondence is something that can make sex extraordinary.

Offer Desires and Expectations

Talk straightforwardly and share your sexual wants. Be transparent about what you need. You would prefer not to utilize this opportunity to be disparaging of your accomplice. Simply attest what you need in the room and what causes you to feel great.

Talk with each other about your desires concerning lovemaking. Bogus or neglected desires can hurt your marriage. If your accomplice is not meeting your desires, convey this prudently and delicately.

Sex in an enduring relationship can extend and turn into a more extravagant encounter. Regardless of how often you have had intercourse to one another, the marvel and stunningness of shared fascination can at present be there.

Make an Arrangement

When life gets occupied and plans are boisterous, plan for sexual experiences with each other. A few people may discover planning unfortunate, yet everything relies upon what you look like at it. You can make arrangements similarly as energizing as unconstrained sex. Being a tease for the day or specifying a "sex date" can construct expectation.

Attempt to set the state of mind ahead of time. If you need to have great sex around evening time, start the foreplay toward the beginning of the day. Tell your accomplice you give it a second thought and are pondering them for the day with notes, messages, writings, calls, embraces, or different coy motions.

Start More Often

Try not to anticipate that your companion should be the just one in your marriage who is liable for sentiment. You both need to assume liability for having a close and fruitful relationship.

Clasp hands and show friendship often. Ladies especially need to feel cherished and associated to have the longing for sex. Set aside a few minutes for date evenings and other novel exercises together and be available to attempting new things!

More Tips for Your Married Sex Life

Even with cautious arranging and certified exertion, you may run into events when sex with your companion doesn't live up to your desires. Remember these tips.

Being crotchety or disregarding your life partner during the day harms your odds of having a positive lovemaking experience that night.

Recollect that sex won't be flawless each time; don't contrast your sex life with the depictions you find in films or on TV.

Perceive that restraint from time to time can be valuable to your relationship. You may find that it constructs expectation and begin to crave each other more. It's about quality before amount.

Take significant consideration of yourself. A stable sex life crosses with your general physical, passionate, and psychological well-being.

CAUSES OF DECLINING SEX DRIVE

It happens to a great deal of folks, however not many of them need to discuss it - particularly when "it" is a low libido. All things considered, virility assumes a major job in our idea of masculinity. There's this thought you should satisfy: "Genuine men are consistently in the state of mind."

Yet, that is not valid. Bunches of men have low sex drive, for a ton of reasons. Furthermore, there are numerous approaches to treat it.

What Causes It?

Any number of things, some physical and some mental. Once in a while it's both.

Physical issues that can cause low libido incorporate low testosterone, physician recommended prescriptions, excessively little or an excess of activity, and liquor and medication use. Mental issues can incorporate wretchedness, stress, and issues in your relationship.

Around 4 out of 10 men over age 45 have low testosterone. While testosterone substitution treatment remains to some degree dubious, it's likewise a typical answer for the issue.

"Supplanting treatment with any of the different testosterones accessible can help libido," says M. Leon Seard, II, MD, a urologist in Nashville, TN. "Additionally, just getting solid can help."

Nobody thing causes low libido. So it's significant to converse with your PCP if you're concerned your sex drive has dropped.

When he makes sense of the causes, he can disclose to you the best strategy, or allude you to another specialist who can.

How Is It Treated?

Contingent upon the reason, potential medicines include:

More beneficial lifestyle decisions. Improve your eating routine, get customary exercise and enough rest, cut down on the liquor, and lessen pressure.

Change to another medicine, if the one you're on is influencing your libido

Testosterone substitution treatment

Directing

Your primary care physician may prescribe treatment if the issue is mental. Much of the time, a low libido focuses to a craving for a closer association with your accomplice - one that isn't sexual, yet at the same time personal. It can assist with talking through these issues with an advisor, either alone or with your accomplice. If the issue is gloom, antidepressants can help. Some of them really bring down your sex drive, however.

Shouldn't something be said about the drugs you may have found in TV and magazine advertisements, similar to Cialis, Levitra, and Viagra? These don't help libido. They assist you with getting and keep erections.

The main concern: Know your body and mention to your PCP what you're feeling. Try not to keep down. That is the main way he'll know whether the foundation of the issue is physical, mental, or both.

Also, the sooner you know, the sooner you can return to feeling like yourself once more.

Low libido portrays a diminished enthusiasm for sexual action.

It's entirely expected to lose enthusiasm for sex now and again, and libido levels fluctuate through life. It's likewise typical for your advantage not to coordinate your accomplice's now and again.

Be that as it may, low libido for an extensive stretch of time may cause worry for certain individuals. It can some of the time be a pointer of a basic wellbeing condition.

Here are a couple of potential reasons for low libido in men.

Low testosterone

Testosterone is a significant male hormone. In men, it's for the most part created in the balls.

Testosterone is answerable for building muscles and bone mass, and for invigorating sperm creation. Your testosterone levels likewise factor into your sex drive.

Ordinary testosterone levels will fluctuate. Be that as it may, grown-up men are considered to have low testosterone, or low T, when their levels fall underneath 300 nanograms for every deciliter (ng/dL), as indicated by rules from the American Urological Association (AUA).

When your testosterone levels decline, your craving for sex likewise diminishes.

Diminishing testosterone is an ordinary piece of maturing. In any case, an uncommon drop in testosterone can prompt diminished libido.

Converse with your primary care physician if you figure this may be an issue for you. You might have the option to take enhancements or gels to expand your testosterone levels.

Prescriptions

Taking certain prescriptions can bring down testosterone levels, which thus may prompt low libido.

For instance, circulatory strain drugs, for example, ACE inhibitors and beta-blockers may forestall discharge and erections.

Different meds that can bring down testosterone levels include:

- chemotherapy or radiation medications for disease
- hormones used to treat prostate malignant growth
- corticosteroids
- narcotic torment relievers, for example, morphine (MorphaBond, MS Contin) and oxycodone (OxyContin, Percocet)
- an antifungal prescription called ketoconazole
- cimetidine (Tagamet), which is utilized for acid reflux and gastroesophageal reflux ailment (GERD)
- anabolic steroids, which might be utilized by competitors to expand bulk
- certain antidepressants

If you're encountering the impacts of low testosterone, converse with your primary care physician. They may encourage you to switch meds.

Fretful legs disorder (RLS)

Fretful legs disorder (RLS) is the wild inclination to move your legs. An examination found that men with RLS are at higher hazard for creating erectile brokenness (ED) than those without RLS. ED happens when a man can't have or keep up an erection.

In the investigation, scientists found that men who had RLS events in any event five times each month were around 50 percent bound to create ED than men without RLS.

Additionally, men who had RLS scenes all the more every now and again were much bound to get barren.

Sadness

Sadness changes all pieces of an individual's life. Individuals with misery experience a decreased or finish absence of enthusiasm for exercises they once discovered pleasurable, including sex.

Low libido is likewise a symptom of certain antidepressants, including:

serotonin-norepinephrine reuptake inhibitors (SNRIs, for example, duloxetine (Cymbalta)

particular serotonin reuptake inhibitors (SSRIs), like fluoxetine (Prozac) and sertraline (Zoloft)

Nonetheless, the norepinephrine and dopamine reuptake inhibitor (NRDI) bupropion (Wellbutrin SR, Wellbutrin XL) hasn't been appeared to decrease the libido.

Converse with your primary care physician if you're taking antidepressants and you have a low libido. They may address your reactions by modifying your portion or having you change to another drug.

Interminable disease

When you're not feeling great because of the impacts of a constant wellbeing condition, for example, ceaseless agony, sex is likely low on your rundown of needs.

Certain ailments, for example, malignant growth, can diminish your sperm creation considers well.

Other ceaseless diseases that can negatively affect your libido include:

- type 2 diabetes
- weight
- hypertension
- elevated cholesterol
- ceaseless lung, heart, kidney, and liver disappointment

If you're encountering a ceaseless disease, talk with your accomplice about approaches to be private during this time. You may likewise think about observing a marriage mentor or sex advisor about your issues.

Rest issues

An examination in the Journal of Clinical Sleep Medicine found that nonobese men with obstructive rest apnea (OSA) experience lower testosterone levels. Thus, this prompts diminished sexual action and libido.

In the examination, analysts found that about 33% of the men who had serious rest apnea additionally had diminished degrees of testosterone.

In another ongoing study in youthful, sound men, testosterone levels were diminished by 10 to 15 percent following seven days of rest limitation to five hours of the night.

The scientists found that the impacts of limiting rest on testosterone levels were particularly clear between 2:00 pm and 10:00 pm the following day.

Maturing

Testosterone levels, which are connected to libido, are at their most elevated when men are in their late adolescents.

In your more established years, it might take more time to have climaxes, discharge, and become excited. Your erections may not be as hard, and it might take more time for your penis to get erect.

In any case, drugs are accessible that can help treat these issues.

Stress

If you're diverted by circumstances or times of high weight, sexual want may diminish. This is because stress can disturb your hormone levels. Your conduits can limit in the midst of pressure. This narrowing limits blood stream and conceivably causes ED.

One investigation distributed in Scientific Research and Essays bolstered the thought that pressure directly affects sexual issues in the two people.

Another investigation of veterans with post-horrendous pressure issue (PTSD) found that the pressure issue expanded their danger of sexual brokenness more than triple.

Stress is difficult to keep away from. Relationship issues, separate, confronting the passing of a friend or family member, budgetary stresses, another infant, or a bustling workplace are only a portion of the life occasions that can incredibly influence the longing for sex.

Stress the executives methods, for example, breathing activities, reflection, and conversing with an advisor, may help.

In one examination, for instance, men who were recently determined to have ED indicated significant improvement in erectile capacity scores subsequent to taking an interest in a 8-week pressure the executives program.

Low confidence

Confidence is characterized as the general conclusion an individual has about their own self. Low confidence, low certainty, and poor self-perception can negatively affect your passionate wellbeing and prosperity.

If you feel that you're ugly, or unwanted, it'll likely discourage sexual experiences. Disliking what you find in the mirror can even make you need to abstain from engaging in sexual relations by and large.

Low confidence may likewise cause tension about sexual execution, which can prompt issues with ED and diminished sexual want.

After some time, confidence issues can bring about bigger psychological wellness issues, for example, gloom, tension, and medication or liquor misuse — all of which have been connected to low libido.

INTIMACY

What is sexual closeness? Sex is a demonstration shared among you and your mate that feels incredible and brings you closer. Closeness is a nearby enthusiastic bond among you and an accomplice. Unite the two and you have a profound association that will strengthen your marriage.

Being close methods something beyond getting physical with your accomplice. Having sexual closeness with your accomplice makes a profound enthusiastic association that adds to an additionally fulfilling sexual bond. Not every person will think that its simple to create sexual closeness and interface with their companion during sex. That is the reason we're taking a gander at 6 different ways you can extend your bond with your accomplice through sexual closeness.

What is sexual closeness?

When used to depict sentimental connections, closeness alludes to a nearby sexual association. Confiding in your life partner and feeling cherished, regarded, agreeable, and safe with them is an enormous piece of sexual closeness. Be that as it may, to characterize sexual closeness, we should have a more critical gander at what happens when accomplices approach.

Individuals let down their passionate watchmen during sex. Likewise, the arrival of the "nestle hormone" oxytocin triggers sentiments of connectedness that permits accomplices to be defenseless and build up trust with each other.

Having sexual closeness implies that you and your accomplice share a unique bond portrayed by a mutual sexy articulation. You see each other on a sexual level that has feeling behind it, rather than it simply being a physical demonstration.

Step by step instructions to associate sincerely during sex

What does being sexually associated mean? It's a physical and passionate bond with your mate. Figure out how to encourage this closeness by associating on a more profound level during sex. Numerous accomplices don't give a lot of consideration to sex and enthusiastic association however them two really supplement one another. Here are the absolute best tips on having a beautiful sexual association and how to make your sex life increasingly sentimental and significant.

1. Setting the stage

Do you need an all the more fulfilling physical and enthusiastic relationship with your accomplice? Who doesn't! One way you can interface more during sex is by making way for closeness. Some extraordinary thoughts for setting the disposition incorporate giving each other back rubs, put on a portion of your preferred erotic music, lighting candles, and clearing your calendars for sex and closeness.

If you're searching for a fast in and out, morning sex before work is your go-to. In any case, if you need to interface profoundly with your accomplice, pick a period where neither one of you will be intruded, for example, in the nights or on ends of the week.

Additionally, turn your telephone off. Nothing ruins sentiment in excess of a cellphone jingle going off out of sight to upset the enthusiastic association during sex.

2. Foreplay and development

One approach to interface during sex is to make a development. Bother your accomplice for the duration of the day with underhanded words, charged instant messages or messages, murmurs of romantic things and love, alongside cautious contacts to get them sincerely associated before the physical demonstration occurs. Working up to the minute will cause it to feel progressively extraordinary when it at last occurs. Feelings during sex run high and keeping up an association can take the experience to an entire different level inside and out. So the response to the ordinary inquiry – "how to be all the more sexually personal with your wife?" lies in sufficient measures of foreplay!

3. Keep in touch

It might feel clumsy from the outset, particularly if you're not used to looking affectionately at your accomplice, however keeping in touch with your mate during personal minutes not just encourages you associating sexually with your accomplice yet additionally assists with strengthening your bond.

This activity can cause you to feel open to your accomplice, which then cultivates sentiments of affection and trust. One investigation done by Kellerman, Lewis, and Laird uncovered that couples who kept in touch with each other detailed uplifted sentiments of adoration, enthusiasm, and general warmth toward their accomplices.

3. Talk during intercourse

What is sexual closeness? It's talking during sex. This doesn't mean you should begin having a discussion about what's for supper later.

There are two incredible roads for talking during sex that you can investigate with your accomplice. Initially, you can have a go at talking shrewd to each other. You can be as realistic or as held as you can imagine with this one. This an incredible method to release your restraints and interface with your words and dreams for getting physically involved with somebody.

You could likewise adopt an a lot better strategy and say romantic things to each other. Mention to your life partner what you like about what you are doing, reveal to them you love them, and state how close you feel to them.

Whatever words you pick, simply recollect that talking during sex is basically an approach to keep your consideration concentrated on each other during these sexually close minutes.

4. Participate in physical touch

How to make sex energetic? All things considered, when being private together don't be reluctant to contact the pieces of each other that aren't erogenous zones. Take a stab at stroking your better half's arms or run your hands through your wife's hair during the demonstration. This will assist you with interfacing on a passionate level and remind you to concentrate on each other during closeness.

5. Deal with one another's enthusiastic needs

One significant piece of a solid relationship is ensuring you are dealing with your life partner's passionate needs just as their physical ones which incorporates closeness and sex. Manufacture trust and show your accomplice regard to help make enthusiastic closeness.

Offer commendations and guarantee your accomplice of your adoration. Be fun loving with one another and have a normal night out on the town. The more associated you are outside of the room, the better your sex life will be. What's more, the less confused you will be about what is close sex. It's actually that straightforward!

6. Snuggle and kiss

Being personal when sex is an incredible method to encourage closeness. You can do this by kissing often. Kissing is an incredible method to construct strain and associate with your accomplice. Kissing is additionally appeared to expand serotonin, which causes you rest better, advance excitement, improve invulnerability, increment oxytocin and dopamine, and abatement stress.

Different approaches to build closeness is to snuggle after sex for a least two or three minutes, spoon before resting, and do a 6-second kiss each prior day going to work.

Sexual closeness happens when you have a sense of security, adored, and excited by your accomplice. There are numerous approaches to intensify your close association with your mate during personal sex. Set up a period where you will be separated from everyone else with your mate without interference, keep in touch during sex, and impart transparently about your physical and passionate needs. Doing this normally will prompt an additionally fulfilling sex life in your marriage.

Closeness. Individuals often mistake it for sex. In any case, individuals can be sexual without being private. Single night rendezvous, companions with advantages, or sex without affection are instances of simply physical acts with no closeness included. They are what they are, however they don't encourage warmth, closeness or trust.

Closeness implies profoundly knowing someone else and feeling profoundly known. That doesn't occur in a discussion in a bar or during a stunning day at the sea shore or even on occasion during sex. It doesn't occur in the main many months of another and energizing relationship. It doesn't create when one individual sustains a relationship more than the other. No. Closeness, similar to fine wine sets aside effort to extend and smooth. It takes delicate dealing with and persistence by completely included. It takes the ability to commit errors and to excuse them for the sake of learning.

Closeness is the thing that a great many people long for yet not every person finds, or rather, makes. Why? Because closeness, genuine closeness with another person, can likewise be startling. Finding a good pace center of a relationship necessitates that the two individuals work through their dread. By visiting and returning to these regions, closeness develops and progresses after some time.

What Intimacy Involves:

Knowing: A really close connection tells the two individuals on the most profound level who they each genuinely are. They have investigated each other's spirit and discovered what something they esteem and acknowledge such a lot of that it can withstand the unavoidable differences that exist between any two people.

Acknowledgment: Neither individual wants to change the other or to change themselves in basic manners. Gracious truly, minor changes consistently happen when individuals suit each other to live respectively. Yet, neither individual from the couple thinks to oneself, "Well – with time, I'll get that person to change what their identity is."

Valuation for differences: Both comprehend that they don't should be totally the equivalent to be close. Actually, some portion of the enjoyment of connections is the disclosure of differences and thankfulness for one another's uniqueness. Finding out about one another's perspectives is viewed as a chance to grow their universes.

Wellbeing: True closeness happens when the two individuals have a sense of security enough to be powerless. There is support for one another's shortcomings and festivity of one another's qualities. The couple has conceded to a meaning of devotion and both have a sense of safety that the other won't abuse that understanding.

Sympathetic critical thinking: Elephants don't come to remain in the "room" of the relationship. Issues are stood up to by the two individuals with affection, empathy and an ability to draw in with whatever issues have come up. The two work to be on a similar group, taking care of an issue, instead of on different groups contending with one another.

Enthusiastic association: Intimacy develops when individuals remain genuinely associated, in any event, when there are issues to explain. It doesn't require that either individual tread lightly or retain what they truly think so as to remain associated.

The most effective method to Nurture Intimacy:

Pick shrewdly: The principal rule for having a close connection is to pick admirably in any case. If being in the relationship with your beau/sweetheart necessitates that you surrender who you truly are, that you generally oblige, or that you roll out crucial improvements to be satisfactory, this individual isn't for you. Much all the more telling is if your accomplice normally charges, faults or bothers you or necessitates that you not remain near different companions. Cut your misfortunes. Get out. Make yourself accessible for somebody who will respect and value you and bolster you for what your identity is.

Show yourselves: As another relationship develops, bit by bit demonstrate yourselves to one another – both the most appealing and the not all that alluring highlights of what your identity is. Be happy to uncover your center convictions, qualities and thoughts to find different's responses. Alternate extremes may at first pull in however they are likewise often the seeds of disappointment as a relationship advances after some time. Investigate your differences and choose if they are fascinating and energizing or major issues. Ensure that your differences don't damage fundamental beliefs for either individual.

Draw a circle: Intimacy necessitates that your relationship with one another is by one way or another different from your associations with every other person. Numerous couples draw the limit around their sexual selectiveness. Others characterize their closeness in different manners. Whatever your choice about devotion, there should be something you both concur is the center of what makes your relationship exceptional, valuable, and extraordinary from all others. Both concur that limit is critical to the point that disregarding it would shake the very establishment of your couple-ness.

Create passionate care: Emotions aren't fortunate or unfortunate. Be that as it may, how we express them can either improve or harm closeness. It's inescapable that every one of you will feel outrage, hurt or disillusionment on occasion, maybe even commonly. Closeness requires learning approaches to communicate those sentiments that are neither threatening nor removing. Work together to find approaches to quiet extreme emotions as opposed to becoming involved with them. Consent to chip away at finding and tending to the base of issues as opposed to detonating or pulling back.

Grasp struggle: Yes, grasp it. Overlooking clash once in a while fills in as a way to closeness. Whatever the contention was about just goes underground, putrefies, and inevitably turns out in ugly and often antagonistic ways. Strife is a sign that there is an issue that should be illuminated. Closeness requires confronting issues with fortitude and with the confidence that the relationship is a higher priority than whatever emergency is going on at the time.

Be the individual you need your accomplice to be: It's anything but difficult to need another person to be understanding, sympathetic, devoted, giving and liberal. It's not all that simple to do it. Closeness necessitates that we do our absolute best to be somebody worth getting physically involved with. It's not important to be flawless at it. It is important to put forth a valiant effort and to be available to criticism when we come up short.

EASY SEX POSITION

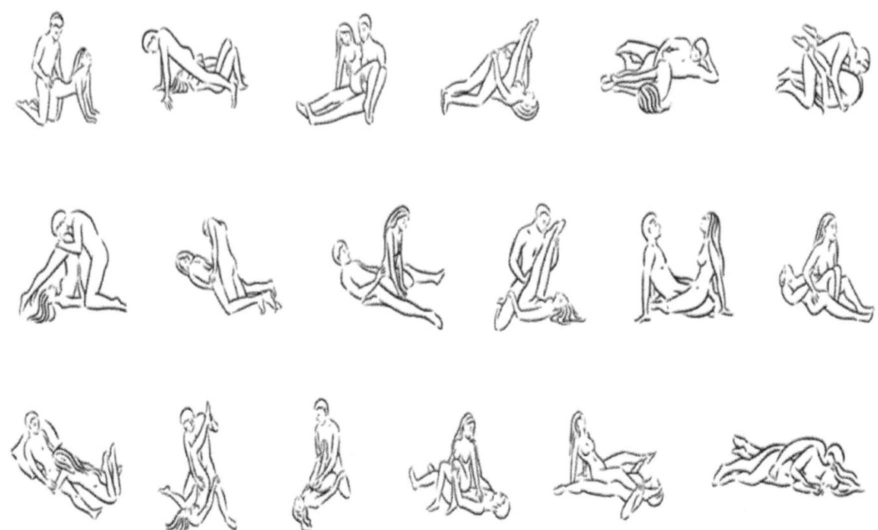

If there's a small piece of you thinking "ouch" during sex, then it's a great opportunity to return to your room methodology. Sex ought to never be awkward... aside from possibly in that divertingly ungainly way.

Regardless of whether position A worked for your past accomplice, your new S.O. will be evidently different. How their own taste lines up with yours will decide agreeable or difficult sex. Truth be told, if one position wasn't so hot last time with accomplice C, it's alright to attempt again with accomplice D. This time, simply join our improved for-solace and-fulfillment sex positions underneath.

With these how-tos, we've kept clitoral incitement (and your pleasure) at the cutting edge. The main prep you have to do — and this is valid before each sort of infiltration with any accomplice — is convey and grease up! Vaginal grease helps significantly lessen contact and inconvenience (and it's flawlessly alright to utilize lube) and prepares for satisfying sex.

1. Sizzling preacher

Relinquish any old recollections of those blameless occasions when fairly cadenced here and there was all you thought about sex. Rather, make another experience of the exemplary minister. Instead of broadening your legs, have your accomplice's legs straddle your body, allowing for shared genital contacting. This works incredible because it isn't subject to estimate yet on the association you and your accomplice have.

2. Sitting on pad top

Take your preferred pad, and spot it underneath your pelvis for expanded help. Curve your knees, bring your pelvis upward, and spread your legs sufficiently separated to take into consideration pushing. What's fabulous about this position is that it permits you to control the profundity of infiltration and advances clitoral incitement.

3. Riding into the nightfall

Take control and jump on top. This position is perfect for some comfortable occasions because it takes into consideration personal kissing and eye staring, and allows you to make the beat you most appreciate. Not exclusively will you have the option to situate your clitoris just as you would prefer and increment sexual joy, yet you can likewise shake your pelvis to and fro to make an agreeable mood.

4. Incline toward me

Discover a divider or table to incline toward. Face one another and pick who will hold each other's butts, and snare their leg around the other individual's leg for help. Animate one another, by scouring your clitoris against your accomplice's private parts, and afterward make an agreeable musicality whereby you're ready to draw your body nearer or away.

5. Side nestle

You can either confront one another, or position yourself to allow section from behind. If you're confronting your accomplice, you can take rule of your sex toy or the penis shaft and make the point and push you want. In the back section position, utilize your rear end to control the speed and have your accomplice stay still, while you move at your own pace and control the profundity.

6. The couple

Pair your preferred situation with self-joy by fusing the manner in which you like to feel great at the same time. If you're utilized to self-animating your clitoris while lying on your back, with or without a sex toy, then do only that while welcoming your accomplice to contact your bosoms or kiss you. Making this pair sensation can be explosive.

7. The bunny

Who said that sex toys are just for solo play? Residue off your preferred vibrator and demonstrate it to your accomplice. Plan to utilize it next time by legitimately applying clitoral incitement while you explore different avenues regarding different positions.

Utilize the different vibration settings to expand your pleasure or bother each other. Take a stab at holding off on climaxing until you can't keep down. The most significant thing, generally, when including another sex toy, is that you both convey about everything without exception – particularly on what feels great to one another.

8. The blacklist

If you've had a go at everything, you're despite everything encountering torment – particularly with infiltration – then it's a great opportunity to blacklist entrance for a tad. To substitute, practice sensate center activities. Maintain the emphasis on developing sexy touch, sexual back rub, and delight rather than execution.

To flavor things up throughout this break, you could check out 69. Just, go on your back and have your significant other's mouth face your private parts, while you discover your mouth to theirs. Set aside the effort to appreciate investigating one another.

When you're an amateur, sex can feel truly overpowering, so there's no disgrace in discovering some simple sex positions to assist you with finding your feet. It requires some investment to realize what you like, what your accomplice loves, and even exactly how things fit together once in a while. What's more, don't kick me off on how to manage your hands if you're on top. I may never get that right. I've simply kind of surrendered.

If you don't know where to begin, simply recollect that one of the most significant things is to back off and permit yourself to unwind. "Perhaps the best activity when your accomplice has constrained sexual experience is to focus on your pace," Tristan Weedmark, worldwide energy represetative for We-Vibe tells Bustle. "There's no motivation to hurry into something in bed that may incite uneasiness. Peruse your accomplice's non-verbal communication and remain aware of how rapidly you're moving." And if you're both new to it that is no issue—you can find what you like together.

So move slowly with places that won't be excessively testing, moves where you can concentrate on making sense of things, and places that vibe cozy, protected and associated. Here are some incredible ones to attempt if you're a novice:

1. Vis-à-vis

Step by step instructions to Do It: Laying on your sides and confronting one another, move marginally higher up on the bed—so your hips are over your partner's. Fold your top leg over them and guide them within you. Lube can help if it's an unbalanced fit.

Why It's Great For Beginners: If you're new, you will be on top of your accomplice to ensure you're both agreeable. This is a cozy position that you can unwind into – with profound entrance.

2. Teacher

Instructions to Do It: If you start in minister, have your accomplice move their hips higher up the bed while you fold your legs over them. This will give you much more incitement than conventional evangelist.

Why It's Great For Beginners: Missionary is an incredible go-to for novices, however this variety is a superior situation for climax. In addition, you're both in an agreeable situation to simply concentrate on one another and ensure you're both getting what you need.

3. On Top (Modified)

Step by step instructions to Do It: Have your accomplice incline toward the divider or a sofa while you straddle them and drop down. For significantly more closeness, they can twist their knees so they're helping prop you up.

Why It's Great For Beginners: On top is an extraordinary position, however a few ladies feel somewhat uncovered or awkward – particularly when they're unpracticed. This permits you to be in charge, however with an increasingly cozy and associated alternative.

4. Doggy

Step by step instructions to Do It: Rest on all fours and spread your legs so your accomplice can bow behind you. You may require your legs further separated or closer together, contingent upon your stature differences.

Why It's Great For Beginners: Even however you're new, you may like greater force. This position lets you try different things with more profound infiltration and leaves a hand free for clit play.

5. Modified Doggy

The most effective method to Do It: Either change from doggy style down onto your elbows, or start by laying on your stomach. A pad under your hips can assist you with finding the correct edge.

Why It's Great For Beginners: If doggy is unreasonably exceptional for you, this is gentler—yet similarly as sexy. It's likewise extraordinary for any murmuring or filthy talk you need to attempt.

6. Spooning

The most effective method to Do It: Lay in the spooning position with your hips over your partner's. Lift your top leg somewhat so your accomplice can enter you. If it's a cumbersome fit, attempt some lube.

Why It's Great For Beginners: Another choice for G-spot incitement, yet this is the most agreeable one. When you get the fit right, you can simply appreciate it.

7. Cowgirl

Step by step instructions to Do It: Once you're feeling progressively good and more certain, you can go for full cowgirl. Straddle your accomplice and guide them inside you. You can generally utilize your hands to help balance.

Why It's Great For Beginners: You can lean forward, back, bob, pound, and so forth. It's an incredible situation for a learner to realize what they like, and it offers extraordinary perspectives and eye to eye connection.

If you're an amateur, there's no disgrace in taking as much time as is needed to make sense of what you like. Move slow and follow what feels better — there's bounty to browse.

INTERMEDIATE SEX POSITIONS

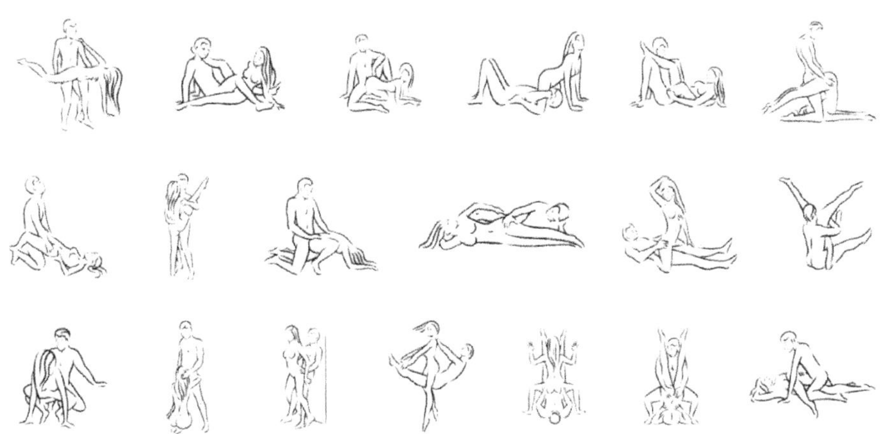

Toward the day's end, sex is much the same as some other game or performing artistry:

The conclusive outcome is just worth the vitality and practice you put into it.

Sex can be out and out enticing, or an all out nap fest – and a great deal of it has to do with the measure of exertion that you and the lady you're with placed into it.

So if you're prepared to change it up a bit, and zest up your sex life... it can mean the difference between exhausting, unremarkable sex, and completely amazing sex.

(I don't think about you, yet I'll take the last mentioned – and as quite a bit of it as I can get, if you don't mind

Sex ought to be something you and your accomplice ceaselessly gain from and improve, so as to keep it crisp, energizing, and pleasant.

So whether you're new to engaging in sexual relations...

Searching for further developed, test, or plain different sex positions...

Or on the other hand searching for different sex positions to drive her wild...

You've gone to the opportune spot.

Amateur Vs. Transitional Vs. Propelled: How To Choose the Right Positions For You

Right now, going to walk you through the best different sex positions for:

Amateurs hoping to ace fundamental sex moves...

Experienced individuals hoping to analyze or get familiar with some new deceives...

Those keen on discovering moves that drive her wild and take her over the edge...

Also, significantly more. I'll show you the 5 best moves for every class, experience what makes them so hot, and disclose how to give them a shot.

In any case, before we start, you may be pondering:

"How would I know if I'm a tenderfoot or further developed?"

Also, at last, I can't answer that – no one but you can genuinely respond to that question for yourself.

Be that as it may, if you aren't sure, my suggestion is to skim through the "Apprentice" positions and proceed onward to the accompanying segments once you feel acquainted with those.

While these moves probably won't work superbly for everybody, there are varieties you can give it a shot and edge alteration suggestions that will assist you with idealizing each position.

Have you previously aced the fundamentals... ?

Or on the other hand perhaps you're simply searching for to a greater degree a test in bed... ?

Maybe you and your better half are needing to explore, yet you don't know precisely where to begin.

These 5 positions will be extraordinary venturing stones into your experimentation with sex. Additionally, huge numbers of them can be performed with props or subjugation methods to kick it up an indent truly.

1) Doggy Style

different-sex-positions-doggy-style

This is an extraordinary situation to evaluate when you first beginning spicing things up...

If you've never attempted this cherished position or if you're hoping to get progressively exploratory, Doggy Style is the ideal spot to begin.

It's an incredible prologue to more unpleasant sex and can be strongly pleasurable for both you and the lady you're with.

To consummate this position, have her bow down on the bed, then lower her chest area so she's on all fours.

Bow or set down behind her and enter her from behind.

Additionally, remember that you will likely need to play with the point after you enter her.

For instance, a 90-degree (opposite) edge of section probably won't feel astounding for her...

Be that as it may, utilizing pads or having her let her head down could help twist her body with the goal that you're entering from an edge she cherishes.

If you've just aced this position or you're hoping to kick things up a score, then Doggy Style is likewise an extraordinary method to begin trying different things with butt-centric sex.

Start with toys first, and change the edge until both of you are agreeable enough to pull out all the stops.

For an additional tad of wrinkle, have a go at riding her while pulling her hair or secures her.

(As a lady, I can reveal to you that the vast majority of us need you to be truly unpleasant with us in bed... here are 3 different ways to do it I guarantee she'll adore.)

15 Different Sex Positions You Haven't Tried Before

2) Spread Eagle

This is an incredible situation to investigate some light BDSM...

If you're truly hoping to flavor up your sex life, there's nothing better than a move that requires some minor subjugation.

The Spread Eagle is an unfathomable situation for anybody keen on dallying with BDSM or simply searching for some additional enjoyment in bed.

To consummate this position, have her rests on her back. Next, have her lift her legs and arms open to question.

If you'd like, you can make it so her legs and arms contact.

What's more, to be significantly kinkier, you can tie her legs and her arms together. Ensure the bunch is tight, yet not very tight to remove her flow.

At last, enter her from above (like Missionary).

This places you in unlimited authority of the circumstance, which is perfect if you're hoping to play with Dominant/Submissive jobs.

Regardless of whether you aren't into BDSM, this position can be amazingly exciting, insofar as there is finished trust among you and your accomplice.

15 Different Sex Positions You Haven't Tried Before

3) Reverse Cowgirl

Bid farewell to preacher with the Reverse Cowgirl

Overjoyed up, rancher!

Put her in the driver's seat with this unbelievable position.

This variety of Girl on Top offers her more authority over the circumstance, while likewise permitting you to loosen up additional. Furthermore, you get an extraordinary view while you're doing it. Falsehood level on your back or at an edge and have her straddle you with the goal that she's confronting your feet. She would then be able to utilize her thighs to swivel and bob here and there.

To make it somewhat more extraordinary and to give her some more influence, twist your knees so she can utilize them to help lift her body here and there.

What's more, if you need to take this position considerably further, have her secure you so you can't do anything aside from lay back and appreciate the ride.

4) Inclined Doggy Style

If you have stairs you're certainly going to need to evaluate this position...

Do you want to try different things with certain edges? This position is ideal for you.

It's one of the most creative modifications to customary Doggy Style and may be exactly what you have to flavor up your sex life.

You'll require stairs to get this going, and it's additionally an extraordinary situation for both vaginal and butt-centric sex — I'll allow you to choose.

To pull it off, have the lady you're with bow on a stair and let her slender forward with her chest area so she's laying on the means over her legs.

Then you do likewise, with the exception of your chest area will lay on hers as you enter her from behind.

It's perhaps the most ideal approaches to make sense of what points drive both of you wild and can be the ideal "entryway tranquilize" to begin trying different things with sex in unusual spots.

5) Wet and Wild

Evaluate this situation for some additional enjoyment in the shower...

You don't need to consolidate shiny new moves into the room to test — rather, have a go at changing your condition.

Shower sex can be a great deal of fun (insofar as you're cautious), so if you're hoping to switch up your sex normal, simply include water.

To be effective at shower sex, ensure you have an amazing silicone-based lube for her and something solid for you to clutch.

You can attempt a standing Doggy Style position where she twists around, or you could likewise take a stab at standing vis-à-vis while you enter her (twist her leg for help).

Trying different things with sex is an enjoyment part of any solid relationship, so don't let the positions accomplish all the work for you.

Take a stab at consolidating messy talk...

Sex toys...

Servitude...

Or on the other hand different props that you both concur will truly help push things to the following super-sexy level.

While sex is typically a ton of good times for the vast majority of us women...

It can in any case be extremely difficult to really have a climax during the deed (regardless of whether what you're doing feels incredibly great).

Nonetheless, while climaxing during sex can be a genuine test for most ladies – it's unquestionably not feasible.

(Like did you realize her climax is 80% almost certain if you can do this to her? It's so cracking simple as well.)

Perhaps the most straightforward ways for a lady to climax through intercourse is by putting her in the driver's seat. Along these lines, she can animate her body the manner in which she needs.

Obviously, there are likewise ways for you to control her developments while additionally taking her breath away.

So if you need to do all that you can to give her the sexual delight she hungers for, have a go at including (at least one) of these sex positions to your arms stockpile.

1) The Fusion

This Fusion position is extraordinary for increasingly extreme climaxes...

This position is somewhat more entangled to pull off, yet it's so worth the exertion.

It offers better development control for her while furnishing you with the best view in the house. 😉

To consummate this position, sit on the bed with your legs spread. Then recline and prop yourself up utilizing the palms of your hands.

From that point, have her sit confronting you between your legs, and prop her decisive advantages over your shoulders. She'll likewise be reclining somewhat and supporting her weight with her palms.

This position permits her to go all over or around and around, giving quicker and increasingly serious climaxes for both of you.

2) The Waterfall

Evaluate this Waterfall strategy for a totally different edge and more profound infiltration...

This position doesn't occur in the shower – rather, it's named after the manner in which it looks.

In addition to the fact that it provides better power over developments for her, yet it additionally guarantees you have probably the best climax of your life.

Give it a shot by laying level on your back (at the foot of the bed).

Gradually slide your take and back off of the bed with the goal that your head and shoulders are on the floor.

Now, your body will be curved in a sort of cascade shape. Next, have her sit on you — from that point, she can squeeze her heels against the edge of the bed and crush and down, moving her hips around and around.

The genuine mystery to this stunt is that the blood in your body is going to race to your head, making your climax considerably more extraordinary than you at any point thought conceivable.

It's additionally phenomenal for her because she can prod you while developing to her own climax.

3) Lowered Reverse Cowgirl

Evaluate this changed form of Reverse Cowgirl... Like Reverse Cowgirl, this move keeps the lady in charge everything being equal.

What makes it different here is that her body will be in a superior situation to really explore her developments all the more decisively — this builds her odds of arriving at climax significantly.

To pull off this position, get into the standard Reverse Cowgirl position.

From that point, have her let herself down to your legs or feet, and she can utilize the palms of her hands and her knees to help bolster her body.

This will offer her better command over her developments, permitting her to hit quite a few spots.

4) Pinball Wizard

Make her climax hard with the Pinball Wizard move..

Did you experience childhood with arcade games? Pinball, maybe?

All things considered, consider this the "grown-up" variant of pinball.

This position gives you control of the circumstance and furthermore makes it simpler to bring the lady you're with to climax.

What's better, it should likewise be possible as unpleasant (or "vanilla") as you need and can be modified in a couple of different ways.

To consummate this position, stoop down on the bed and have her lay before you.

Lift her advantages and grasp her thighs to help push in and out.

You can modify this somewhat by having her ribbon her lower legs around your neck or over your shoulders.

This hot position feels naughtier than most... but on the other hand it's an incredible method to give her a simple climax (the chances of a lady having a climax are expanded whenever her legs are noticeable all around).

5) Magic Mountain

Make sex into an enjoyment ride with this Magic Mountain move...

The "Enchantment Mountain" doesn't simply stable like an enjoyment ride at an entertainment mecca... it likewise feels astonishing.

It makes it similarly simple for both you and the lady you're with to control your developments — and what's more, it makes it route simpler for her to get done with during sex.

Put a pile of cushions on the floor. Have the lady you're with hang over the pads and "unwind" into them.

Her back should normally curve.

You need to lay on her back so your chest is "stuck" to her. Your arms ought to be on hers.

Then enter her from behind, much the same as doggie style.

You can now securely go "full scale" with your pushes, since she has a lot of cushioning.

Be that as it may, it likewise gives her an expanded feeling of association and skin-to-skin contact.

The best part about this move is that there's a mutual feeling of sexual control.

By the day's end, sex ought to be a good time for both you and the lady you're with... and these positions ought to absolutely assist you with arriving.

In any case, I have to admit — there is one more thing you can do to ensure you're really great she's at any point had.

ADVANCED SEX POSITIONS

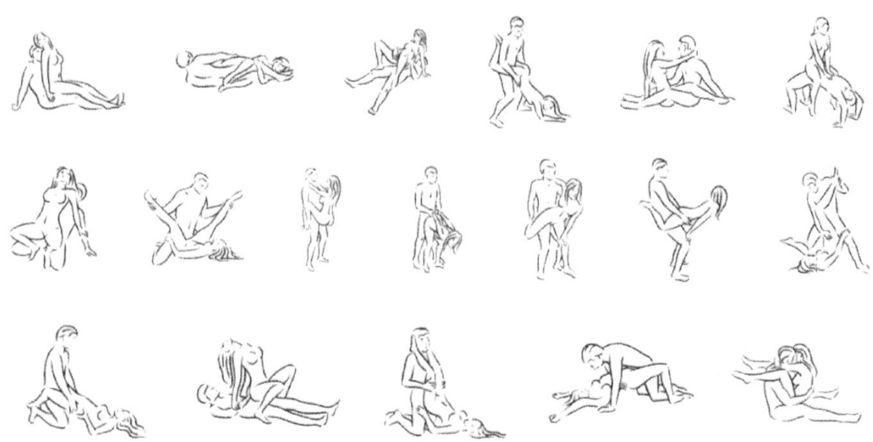

Sex resembles frozen yogurt; we as a whole have our preferred flavor. When we've discovered the one that that fulfills us without fail, we stay with it. Hello, why fix anything if it's not broken? Yet, let's be honest, treats 'n' cream after a long time after night will have even the most committed client desiring another spoonful to appreciate.

Regardless of whether we're discussing tidbits or sex positions, it's acceptable to attempt new things. As per an ongoing sex study, the best indicator of long haul sexual fulfillment for couples was an ability to take a stab at something new, and sex positions were at the highest priority on the rundown.

Indeed, while you may have aced preacher and doggy-style back in your 20s, there's in no way like the rush of playing with some wild moves together. Attempting new, progressively brave sex positions won't just assist you with enduring longer, yet will likewise stretch out the excursion to peak, making those last minutes such a great amount of better for you both.

Be cautious, however — these positions are not for fledglings.

Feline (COITAL ALIGNMENT TECHNIQUE)

For ladies that experience difficulty arriving at climax through intercourse alone, the Coital Alignment Technique (otherwise called the CAT position) can be The One. What's more, what man wouldn't like to be the person who gets her there?

To nail the CAT position, start off in preacher and, after infiltration, slide your pelvis a couple of inches higher than expected. Keep your body level against hers and as opposed to moving in and out, concoct and down — the key here is to be pelvis-to-pelvis so the base of your penis can invigorate your accomplice's clitoris. She should fold her legs over you, either keeping her hips still or turning them for more noteworthy contact. If you're experiencing difficulty hitting the spot, have a go at setting a cushion under her butt or making a roundabout movement with your hips. Snatching the headboard and consolidating pulls with hip pushes assists with your point and lets you infiltrate her more profound. To really open this current position's latent capacity, reach your pelvic bone as the consistent, shaking movement brings you both to an incredible peak. Go on, rock her reality.

THE SITTING V

Despite the fact that the Sitting V is an entirely clear situation for men, it requires a specific measure of adaptability from your accomplice. What amount? Consider this: if she can't contact her toes in a forward overlap, it probably won't be the correct decision. To pull it off, have your sweetheart sit on a high seat or ledge confronting you, while you face her with your feet spread separated. Modify the separation until your pelvis adjusts flawlessly with hers before having her place her lower legs over your shoulders, moving her body into an 'Angular' shape against you. She would then be able to recline, utilizing the divider or her arms as help, or pull herself closer to you by folding her arms over your neck (Although this alternative builds the stretch on her hamstrings)... If you need to help make the position increasingly agreeable for her, have a go at supporting her middle with your hands around her back.

This position permits you to infiltrate your accomplice profoundly and control the beat and profundity of your developments, letting you set the tone to the peak. The capacity for ground-breaking pushing, joined easily of execution, can make this a seriously animating posture.

THE SCISSORS

Not simply held for young lady on-young lady activity, scissoring can truly hit the spot for hetero couples too. Begin sitting up on a delicate surface with your legs collapsed in a topsy turvy "V" while she lays on her side with her legs open and knees somewhat twisted; your lower parts should meet an a nearly right point. Spot your upper leg over her lower leg and your lower leg underneath hers, then shift sufficiently close to enter her. In spite of the fact that it might be dubious to locate the ideal situation from the start, when you get it, the laid-back yet extreme incitement will keep you and your darling returning for additional.

The Scissors probably won't permit a lot of scope of movement, yet don't be debilitated — there's a lot of joy to be had for all! The situating of your entwined legs gives your accomplice persistent clitoral incitement, while the shallow pushes energize the nerve endings on the leader of your penis, taking into consideration an electrifying form to climax.

Face-Sitting

Not unreasonably you need a reason to go downtown, however face-sitting presents an agreeable, low-sway approach to give your woman unadulterated euphoria. If you wind up requiring a minute to regain some composure between positions, or are feeling — ahem — over-animated, lay back and put the attention on the main thing: her pleasure. Have your accomplice straddle your head, being certain to leave you a couple of crawls of breathing room, before she settles in and you get down to business. Odds are she'll require something to clutch, since you'll be doing such a great job causing her to squirm with joy. A divider or bedpost proves to be useful for balance, while tucking her calves under your shoulders includes additional steadiness.

This posture is useful for those as yet culminating their tongue strategy, as it permits the face-sitter to control the position and force more definitely than if she was laying on her back. Also, most definitely... If the view from this edge wasn't sufficient to make you go, her butt and hips are in simple reach for a crush of enjoyment.

SIDEWAYS 69

It resembles I generally state, once in a while you have to give a little to get a bit. However, there's definitely no explanation that you can't give and get at the equivalent, isn't that so? That is the reason 69 is such a fan-most loved in the room, because it permits us to furnish a band together with consistent delight without sacrificing our very own moment. Also, when you turn 69 on its side, you can give for such a long time you could conceivably be blessed sainthood.

Start by laying on your side confronting your accomplice, with your head toward her feet and the other way around. Next, twist your top leg to frame a triangle, with your knee pointing at the roof, putting the top foot level on the bed and supporting yourself on your elbow for balance. Contingent upon your stature and size, you may need to modify the good ways from your accomplice to advance access to their genitals. Despite the fact that it's substantially less famous than customary 69, this sideways variety takes out potential neck-hurts and opens up your hands to participate in the pleasuring, in addition to it's often increasingly agreeable and less unbalanced to hold for an all-inclusive timeframe. Cheerful 69ing!

Cascade

If you're similar to most couples, there are numerous evenings you likely would prefer not to get off the lounge chair — so why not get off on the sofa? The Waterfall is a minor departure from the famous Cowgirl position, yet sneaks up all of a sudden. Start by laying on the lounge chair or bed with your head close to the edge and your young lady on you, however as opposed to riding you from her knees, she'll have to recline and shift her weight to her feet. When she has the position down, crawl toward the edge of the bed or lounge chair, letting your head and shoulders slide off onto the ground while your hips stay raised. If you're on a lounge chair, wrap your legs over the rear of the situate or basically let your knees fall open. From here, your accomplice has unlimited oversight over the speed, profundity and force of her gyrations, also a free hand to use as she wishes — clitoral incitement, anybody?

There are a few different ways to execute this posture: You can either utilize it as a scaffold while working to climax, or moving into it directly before the enormous finale. In any case, this position will make the blood hurry to your head (and your other head) for a dangerous peak. (Presently you'll comprehend why it's known as the Waterfall).

G-SPOT SEX POSITIONS

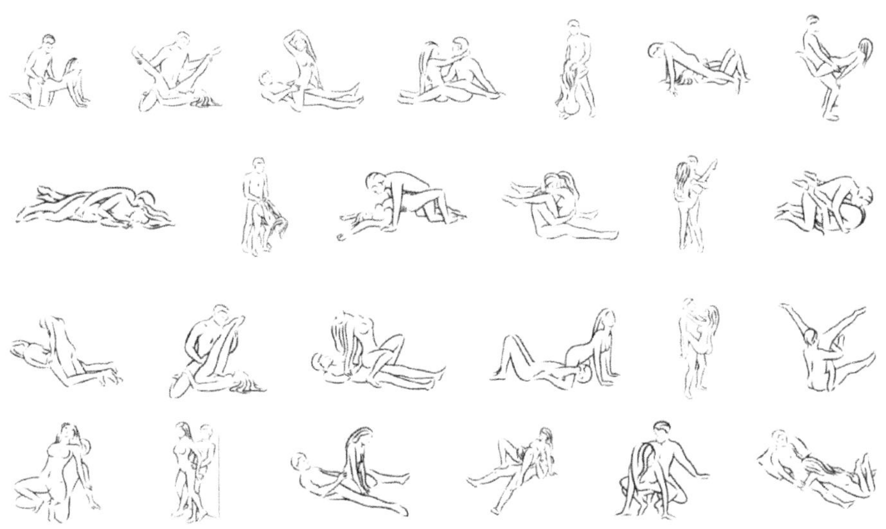

If a lady's life structures were Disney World (not to make Disney unusual or anything...), her clitoris would be the Magic Kingdom—the headliner where all the enjoyment and firecrackers occur. What's more, her G-detect, a little hotspot more profound inside her, ahem, "park," would be Epcot: unquestionably worth a visit, however marginally less energizing all alone.

Why? The G-spot climax is, miserable to state, less dependable than the clitoral kind—yet it's very enchanted if you're ready to arrive (or even better, experience both without a moment's delay, through a mixed climax).

Speedy life systems exercise: Your G-spot is quite of the entire structure of your clitoris, which stretches out three to five creeps inside you along the vaginal waterway. (Get your full Female Anatomy 101 here.)

While everybody's G-spot is in a different, um, spot (sorry to be muddled), it's normally situated around a few creeps inside your vagina along the front divider, says Sari Cooper, certified sex advisor and chief of the Center for Love and Sex in New York City. (Since blood stream to the territory makes it swell, the more stirred you are, the simpler it is to discover.)

"Few out of every odd lady will have a G-spot climax, and that is absolutely ordinary," says Cooper. In any case, if you're ready to have one, you'll feel a surge that is different from the back rub actuated clitoral peak.

Obviously, you won't know until you attempt—and these 10 master endorsed sex positions to animate your G-spot are the primo method to do as such. Most dire outcome imaginable, you end up with a night of super-hot sex. Not a terrible incidental award, if you ask me...

1. The Soft Serve

This position gives the ideal point to his penis to arrive at that front divider where your G-spot is, says Cooper. Have him focus on that, or lean forward more and propel yourself again into him to arrive, she says. What makes this move far superior? You both have simple clit get to, so utilize your hands or a vibe to have a clitoral climax first—that blood stream will cause the G-spot to expand, making it bigger and simpler to go after a second huge O.

Do It: Get into the spooning position with him as the enormous spoon. Bring your knees up somewhat and have him enter you from behind.

2. Young lady On Fire

This sex position offers an opportunity in point that helps focus on your G-spot significantly progressively—in addition to gives you command over the speed and profundity of pushes. Gracious, and not in vain: Your accomplice has simple access to your clitoris so that you can take a shot at that subtle mixed climax.

Do It: This position is much the same as cowgirl, yet with a wind. Get on top and have your accomplice enter you. Then, recline and place your hands on the bed for help, making a 45-degree edge with your accomplice's legs.

3. G-Whiz

If the name alone is anything but an obvious hint, this sex position is amazing because when you raise your legs, it limits the vagina and helps focus on your G-spot. Need to raise the stakes? Request that your accomplice begin shaking you in a side-to-side or here and there movement. That ought to carry his penis into direct contact with your G-spot.

Do It: Lie back with your legs laying on every one of your accomplice's shoulders.

4. The Snake

This variant of doggy style offers a superior edge to arrive at that front divider, says Cooper. Furthermore, despite the fact that he's accountable for the development here, you can change the edge by raising your hips sequential (or tossing a cushion under them, if you like). You'll adore the profound entrance and cozy attack of him inside you (as will he).

Do It: Lie down on your stomach, and have your accomplice rests on you and slide in from behind.

5. Turn around Scoop

This sexy position has all the advantages of spoon, yet with more exposure. Also, by utilizing shallow pushes, your accomplice has a decent possibility of arriving at your G-spot. Furthermore, you can pound your clit against his pelvis, making for that desired mixed climax.

Do It: Lie down on your sides confronting one another, and get in an agreeable position.

6. Well, Cowgirl

Who doesn't adore young lady on top? You're in control, so move (ricochet, swivel, pound) as you decide to make that G-spot climax occur. Have a go at holding your lower back curved, which will acquire that O closer reach.

Do It: Straddle him, looking ahead, and twist back marginally while clutching his thighs for help.

7. Great Doggy

This position for all intents and purposes ensures G-spot incitement, since it's practically unthinkable for him not to infiltrate profound. Reward: From this position, he can likewise invigorate your bosoms or your clit to amp up your excitement, which builds blood stream to your G-spot.

Do It: Get on your lower arms with your butt noticeable all around. Have your accomplice bow behind you and enter you from behind.

8. The Wheelbarrow

Do you want to make things intriguing? Attempt this hot standing-sex position that will hit your G-spot like a flash. If you get worn out, all great, young lady essentially lay on a table or the side of the bed to offer your arms a reprieve.

Do It: Get on all fours and have your accomplice get you by the pelvis. Then hold his midsection with your thighs.

9. The Big Dipper

With this sex position, you get the more profound entrance and G-spot incitement of doggy, while as yet having the option to look. Have your accomplice rub your clit as he pushes for extra ooooomph.

Do It: Lie on your correct side; your accomplice stoops, straddling your correct leg and twisting your left leg around his left side.

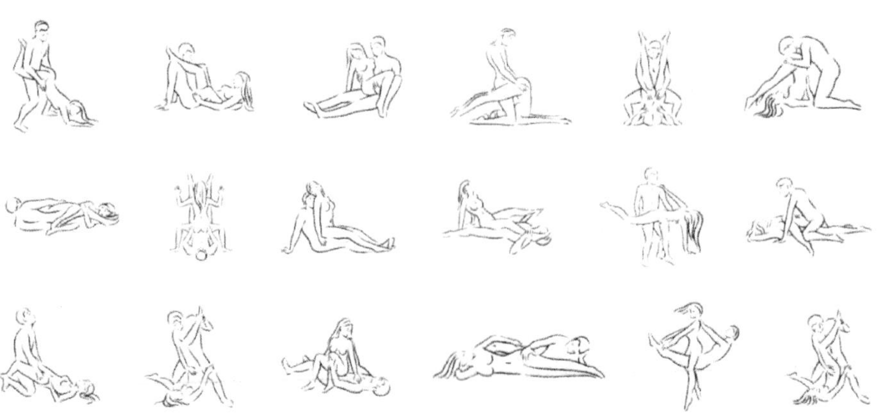

10. The Gee-Shell

This sex position is hot-hot-hot! The perspectives, the points, the...flexibility— by what means can you both not get off? If he "rides low"— a.k.a. doesn't concentrate such a great amount on crushing his pubic bone against your clitoris—the leader of his penis will legitimately invigorate your G-spot. For clitoral activity, go to work with your (advantageously) free hands.

Do It: Lie back with your legs raised as far as possible up and your lower legs crossed behind your own head (or anyway far you can contact them), then have him enter you from a teacher position.

The way to fair sex is cleared with reiteration. Except if "average" is the sort of sex you need to have, it's essential to keep blending things up, giving things a shot and moving toward things from new edges. When it comes to oral sex, you have such huge numbers of different chances to investigate your accomplice's body. Why squander them on the regular old, regular old? Here are several oral sex positions intended to give you a different take on mouth lovin'. With three positions intended to please bands together with penises (fellatio positions) and three positions intended to please cooperates with vaginas (cunnilingus positions), there's a touch of something for everybody! Appreciate!

Hangin' Back (otherwise known as The Deepthroat Position)

If You're Giving It: This is maybe, strategically, the best situation from which to accomplish the subtle deepthroat. It places the mouth and throat into one long queue, empowering you to all the more effectively take a greater amount of your accomplice into your mouth. Because your accomplice has such a great amount of opportunity to move here, you need to utilize your hands to control the movement and keep things agreeable for you. Loosen up the throat and appreciate the vibe of balls on your eyelids! ;-)

If You're Getting It: If you are accepting right now mindful that you may need to stoop, squat or in any case modify your stature to agree with your accomplice's mouth. Likewise, be touchy and mindful so as not to gag your accomplice. It's a smart thought to watch a "tap out" hand signal that demonstrates when your accomplice needs a break.

The Intense Headrest

If You're Giving It: Here's another acceptable one. Here, your accomplice lays on one side and lifts the top leg. You place your head between his legs and the remainder of your body behind his, with the goal that your head lays on his thigh. Your accomplice lays back while you find a good pace. This position gives you liberated access to the penis and gonads and extraordinary points to truly get into it. You can even fold your arms over his legs for more influence (charm! charm!).

If You're Getting It: If you are accepting right now can simply lie back and appreciate it. Or then again, have a go at coming to back with your top arm to contact your accomplice.

The Mellow Headrest

If You're Giving It: Here's one that is fun - yet somewhat more smooth. Your accomplice accept a similar situation as in the extraordinary headrest, above, however this time when you place your head between his legs you flip the entire thing around! Your legs will wind up close to your accomplice's face and you will, by and by, lay your head on his lower thigh. This position is better for taking things a little more slow.

If You're Getting It: If you are accepting right now, accomplice's body is in that spot before you! That implies you have incredible access for manual incitement.

For the Ladies

Woman Godiva

If You're Giving It: Get your woman darling to jump on and have a good time with this position. Lay back (maybe with a cushion propping your head up marginally) and have your accomplice bow and straddle your face. Right now, can offer more incitement by moving your head (not simply the mouth) here and there and side to side as you utilize your tongue.

If You're Getting It: If you are accepting right now can get into a "riding" movement if both you and your accomplice are agreeable. Know about your accomplice's capacity to inhale however. This is another acceptable time to utilize a "tap-out" signal.

Laid Back Loving

If You're Giving It: Just like in the Lady Godiva, you find a good pace with a pad (right now two, neck bolster will be significant here), propping your head up while your accomplice lies face up on your gut with her legs on either side of your head.

If You're Getting It: If you are accepting right now sure that you bring yourself sufficiently close to your accomplice's mouth with the goal that the person in question doesn't need to strain to contact you. Then, simply lay back and appreciate.

Glad Doggy

If You're Giving It: I realize that huge numbers of you like the doggy style sex position. This is a simple oral situation with comparative posing. Have your accomplice jump on all fours confronting endlessly from you with a slight curve in her back and her knees spread wide. This position will permit you to handily get to your accomplice's whole genital district and play with points and ways to deal with find what feels best. You can likewise reach advance and animate your accomplice's bosoms right now.

If You're Getting It: If you are accepting right now can bring down your chest right to the bed/floor/counter/landing area in order to make an even mineral open plot for your hips.

FIFTH BOOK: Kama Sutra

THE SPIRITUALITY OF LOVE

Individuals do insane things when it comes to adore. Some flee from home, others remain in a damaging relationship for the sake of affection, some quit their vocation because their adoration directed in this way, thus considerably more. The vast majority guarantee they are enamored however in actuality, they have no clue what the significance of genuine, profound love is. In certain connections, they are driven by fixation, envy, and terrorizing of their mate. They stalk their life partners wherever they go, they truly and intellectually misuse them, all for the sake of adoration. A few people go to the degree of ensuring their accomplices don't have any companions. That isn't a meaning of adoration; it is a fantasy of affection. The significance of profound love is when you can keep up your independence, in spite of the sentiment of enthusiasm. You can adore without applying any principles to one another. This is unequivocal love. It doesn't make a difference that your companion is revolting, shorter than you, or he snickers in a bothering way. You will adore that person the manner in which the person is. You will cherish all the blemishes the individual depicts and not reprimand them. Numerous individuals apply conditions in their connections, asserting they love one another. For example, you tell your life partner you love him when he gets you something. In otherworldly love, it resembles a spell that has been given occasion to feel qualms about you. You value your significant different as the individual in question is - no condition applies. You love him where it counts and you simply know it in your heart. If you ever wind up in such a circumstance, that is profound love. The following are a few rules to assist you with realizing you are genuinely enamored.

1. You Communicate With Each Other With Ease

In each relationship, correspondence is the way to building a more grounded association. Couples must chat with other often and they should be in the same spot. If you can converse with your companion easily, he won't just tune in yet will likewise have sympathy for the current circumstance. You feel increased in value, you are regarded, and the greater part of all, no judgment is applied. Your companion underpins you completely in the entirety of your undertakings. In such cases, most couples appreciate what they have while it keeps going. They appreciate each other's conversation and they normally search for private space to talk constantly. When one individual is talking, the other is listening acutely. No interferences, no thinking of different alternatives. You are both there for one another and bolster each other while being infatuated. An association in profound love is paid attention to very.

2. Uniformity Applies In Spiritual Love

A great many people don't have the foggiest idea about the meaning of uniformity in a relationship. It implies when two individuals interface and they chose to live respectively, jobs are characterized consequently. You can recognize each other's abilities and regard each other enough to let them do something amazing in your relationship. In each relationship, obligations come naturally. In profound love, you realize who is better at dealing with a specific part of your lives together. Trust applies in such a circumstance where you let your life partner start to lead the pack with no preference or judgment. This doesn't make either the individual in the couple lesser people, it just makes them more infatuated with one another.

3.You Are Attracted To Your Spouse

The vast majority don't have the foggiest idea what fascination implies. Some get pulled in to an individual because of their looks, how they dress, how rich they are, in addition to other things. Otherworldly love is when you need to interface with the individual, mind-wise, body-wise, and to the spirit. You need to be near the individual constantly. When you are as one, you feel an enthusiasm that you have never felt. It resembles an affection spell that has been provided reason to feel ambiguous about you. You are overcome with the energy and yet, you can remain rational. Your independence is as yet unblemished. Besides, there is a whole other world to life other than being diverted by desire.

4. You Find Comfort in Each Other's Company

In profound love, there are no desires from one another, no sprucing up for the other. You simply present yourself as you seem to be. When you are enamored with one another, you feel that you can vanquish the world together. You don't see anything enormous under the sun. You experience happiness when you are as one and you don't scrutinize each other's dedication. Just you two comprehend your association. The manner in which you feel for one another has no simple definition. You simply feel content and your life will have an importance. In many connections, you will discover individuals addressing themselves. They don't believe their judgment and more often than not they rationalize to part. Others go through years seeking their accomplice and not making any genuine duty since they discover imperfections in each other. In otherworldly love, nothing of the sort applies. You love your companion as the individual in question seems to be. You value them for who they truly are. There are no butterflies or second-thinks about when you are as one.

5. In Spiritual Love, There Is No Hurry

Society expects that when there is an association with the one you love, no time ought to be squandered, and you ought to rapidly make courses of action for your future together. Nonetheless, in otherworldly love, nothing of the sort is normal. Couples appreciate each other organization; they leave the destiny of their association to Mother Nature. You don't address if your life partner is the correct individual, if your companion going to be deeply inspired by another, etc. You heed your gut feelings that all will turn out fine and dandy. In profound love, you realize you are under this adoration spell together regardless of what occurs. The manner in which you see the world is the manner in which your mate sees it as well. You associate well with your sweetheart and offer energy.

6. Spiritual Love Promotes Growth

When you interface with somebody and you promise to live respectively, you hope to develop in all ways, particularly self-improvement. Your mate ought to be allowed to tell you your blemishes and you should take them decidedly. Tune in to your companion's recommendation. If somebody cherishes you, you ought not anticipate that the person in question should misdirect you. We can't accomplish self-improvement if our mates don't make some noise about our slip-ups. In profound love, you don't underestimate your mate nor do you consider him to be her as an apparatus to bring home the bacon. This is an extraordinary open door for you to encounter the genuine delight of being enamored.

7. Spiritual Love Does Not Let You Settle for Anything

As an individual, you are qualified for affection life, follow your interests, love a specific lifestyle, to be regarded and cherished. Your life partner ought to likewise esteem the things you love. The person in question ought not direct the manner in which you live. Your adoration ought to figure out how to join their necessities into yours. You should live in amicability and have the option to regard one another. These days, most duties are the inverse. Individuals settle for significantly less. They let their mates direct their method for living and have no common regard in the responsibility, all for the sake of "adoration".

8. Spiritual Love Enables You to Separate Fact from Feelings

In a responsibility resulting from affection, you will have a couple of battles about the years. Yet, that doesn't mean you have an awful relationship or your life partner loathes you. You will blow up at a portion of the remarks the person makes. Rather than misquoting one another, you ought to figure out how to work it out. Let your life partner clarify what the person in question implied.

9. In Spiritual Love, Couples Connect

Individuals in affection look at one another without flinching as they talk. Most customary couples talk for it. Some even talk with their back to their life partner. All things considered, couples who get each other are alright with confronting one another while taking. They can sit opposite one another at a table and speak with their eyes as it were. Who might not think they are under an affection spell? This shows how agreeable they are with one another and that certainty encompasses their adoration.

10. Spiritual Love Makes You Long For the Future

Each relationship differs from the others from numerous points of view. When two perfect partners love each other profoundly, they don't feel worn out on one another no problem at all. The fervor may blur with time, yet interest remains. You will cherish each other increasingly more with spending years. You are two people who have different qualities, however living respectively will empower both of you to investigate each other to the fullest as you age with time. Some case they began to look all starry eyed at from the start sight, however it requires significant investment and development to understand that you profoundly love your companion and that living without the person in question would be unfulfilling. Moreover, everyone might want a chance to develop old with their cherished one. These days, sweethearts settle for much less. They essentially need to profit by one another since they have no better choice. When they discover another person they feel an association with, they go separate ways as opposed to giving their adoration a possibility. Genuine affection requires some investment and tolerance. Indeed, even in the blessed writings of different religions, otherworldly love applies. To summarize everything, profound love is unqualified love that has no limits. It gives significance and significance to your life. Everybody wishes to encounter this sort of affection at one point in life. It is an awesome thing that can't be contrasted with some other inclination on the planet. It is elusive unequivocal love except if you practice some persistence. Couples who have a profound love are more joyful, they see one another, and they battle less. If you are in a profound love, give it your best since no one can really tell when it will end. Gain from one another and acknowledge what both of you have. You are more fortunate than others because you have encountered profound love and you know its definition.

INCREASE SEXUAL PASSION

Jason and Kendra have been hitched for a long time and have three kids. The vast majority of their discussions are about work, tasks, their child's exercises, and everyday parts of their stale marriage.

Kendra puts it like this: "I love Jason, yet the energy simply isn't there any longer."

When Kendra drops this stunner, Jason reacts, "I thought we were doing approve, I truly did. Despite the fact that we don't engage in sexual relations much any longer, it just appears to be a stage we're experiencing. I don't have any energy left when I hit the bed around evening time."

Apparently, Kendra and Jason were energetic during the early long periods of their marriage. Nonetheless, in the course of the most recent couple of years, their sex life has dwindled and they once in a while get to know each other without their kids. Kendra searches out Jason for sexual closeness and Jason often pulls away.

As indicated by specialists, the most widely recognized explanation couples lose their enthusiasm for one another and quit being sexually cozy is a follower distancer design that creates after some time. Dr. Sue Johnson identifies the example of interest pull back as the "Dissent Polka" and says it is one of three "Evil presence Dialogs." She clarifies that when one accomplice gets basic and forceful, the other often gets guarded and far off.

Dr. John Gottman's exploration on a large number of couples found accomplices that stall out right now the initial hardly any long periods of marriage have in excess of a 80% possibility of separating in the initial four to five years.

Encourage Emotional Intimacy

A decent sexual relationship is based on passionate closeness and closeness. As such, if you're planning to improve your physical relationship, you have to deal with your enthusiastic association initially. Concentrate on addressing your accomplice's needs and imparting your own needs in an adoring, deferential way.

In The Science of Trust, Dr. Gottman clarifies that couples who need to revive their energy and love need to turn towards one another. Rehearsing enthusiastic attunement can assist you with remaining associated in any event, when you oppose this idea. This implies moving in the direction of each other by indicating compassion, rather than being cautious. The two accomplices need to discuss their emotions as far as positive need, rather than what they needn't bother with.

As indicated by Dr. Gottman, communicating a positive need is a formula for progress for both the audience and the speaker because it passes on grievances and solicitations without analysis and fault. Dr. Gottman says, "This requires a psychological change based on what's up with one's accomplice to what one's accomplice can accomplish that would work. The speaker is truly saying, 'This is what I feel, and what I need from you.'"

Revive Sexual Chemistry

During the early period of marriage, numerous couples scarcely surface for oxygen because of the energy of experiencing passionate feelings for. Shockingly, this merry state doesn't keep going forever. Researchers have found that oxytocin (a holding hormone) discharged during the underlying phase of captivation makes couples feel euphoric and turned on by physical touch. It really works like a medication, giving us quick rewards that predicament us to our sweetheart.

Clasping hands, embraces, and delicate touch are incredible approaches to certify your affection for your accomplice. Physical warmth makes way for sexual touch that is centered around joy. Sex advisor and teacher Dr. Micheal Stysma suggests that you set an objective of multiplying the period of time you kiss, embrace, and utilize erotic touch if you need to improve your marriage.

Sexual fascination is difficult to keep up after some time. For example, Kendra and Jason need enthusiasm because they are reluctant to surrender control and show defenselessness. Accordingly, they maintain a strategic distance from sex and seldom contact one another. Sex specialist Laurie Watson says, "Most sexual concerns originate from a relational battle in the marriage."

Here are 10 hints to bring back the enthusiasm in your marriage:

1. Change your example of starting sex

Possibly you are denying your accomplice or going ahead excessively solid. Abstain from censuring one another and stop "habitual pettiness." Mix things up to end the force battle. For instance, distancers might need to work on starting sex all the more often and followers attempt to discover approaches to tell their accomplice "you're sexy," in unobtrusive ways while keeping away from investigate and requests for closeness.

2. Clasp hands all the more often

As indicated by creator Dr. Kory Floyd, clasping hands, embracing, and contacting can discharge oxytocin creating a quieting uproar. Studies show it's additionally discharged during sexual climax. Moreover, physical friendship diminishes pressure hormones – bringing down every day levels of the pressure hormone cortisol.

3. Permit strain to construct

Our cerebrums experience more delight when the expectation of the prize continues for quite a while before we get it. So take as much time as is needed during foreplay, share dreams, change areas, and make sex progressively sentimental.

4. Separate sexual closeness from schedule

Plan closeness time and abstain from discussing relationship issues and family errands in the room. Sexual excitement falls when we're diverted and focused.

5. Cut out time to go through with your accomplice

Attempt an assortment of exercises that bring you both delight. Have some good times seeking and work on being a tease as an approach to touch off sexual want and closeness. Dr. Gottman says that "everything positive you do in your relationship is foreplay."

6. Concentrate on friendly touch

Offer to give your accomplice a back or shoulder rub. Individuals partner foreplay with sexual intercourse, however warm touch is a ground-breaking approach to show and revive energy regardless of whether you are not a sensitive feely individual.

7. Work on being all the more sincerely helpless during sex

Offer your deepest wishes, dreams, and wants with your accomplice. If you dread passionate closeness, think about taking part in individual or couple's treatment.

8. Keep up a feeling of interest about sexual closeness

Trial with better approaches to carry joy to one another. Take a gander at sex as a chance to find a workable pace accomplice better after some time.

9. Change the sort of sex you have

Have delicate, adoring delicate, private, and profoundly suggestive sex. Separate the daily schedule and attempt new things as sexual needs change.

10. Focus on sex

Set the mind-set for closeness before TV or work dulls your enthusiasm. A light dinner alongside your preferred music and wine can make way for incredible sex.

BEFORE AND AFTER SEX

We comprehend what to do before sex. What's more, we comprehend what to do during sex. However, shouldn't something be said about after sex? Truly, much the same as the key to being pre-coitally beguiling—and knowing precisely what moves and when to pull in things—the minutes after sex are similarly as significant. Truth be told, as indicated by ladies and sex specialists that we talked with, most men ignore reasonable items, open doors for association, and neglected... needs. What follows is an a master endorsed plan for the day to keep in your room consistently. Fight the temptation to drop after your climax and fuse it into your sex life. You'll be happy that you did—and all the more critically, she will be as well. And keeping in mind that you're grinding away, be certain you're staying away from the 11 things men ought to never at any point do after sex.

1Clean Up.

Sex can be a chaotic business. There's nothing more disgraceful than not offering to clean the sex-related goo from your accomplice's body and prompt environment. Your co-sexer may really like the idea of thriving in your very own marinade making and decrease your offer yet a semen-in-the-eye situation should be managed detail and, thus, it's a strong plan to have some tidy up accessories close within reach. A few tissues or flushable purifying materials are extraordinary to have around and you'll get distraught extra focuses if you return running into the room with a hot towel—the kind of thing that you're given when eating in a sushi eatery. Notwithstanding being set up with a towel, prepare for a major night by learning The Single Best Way To Boost Your Sex Appeal.

2Pee.

You'll have no uncertainty seen that numerous ladies try utilizing the restroom not long after sex is finished and it's often because they need to reduce the probability of getting a urinary tract disease or UTI. It's less regular for a person to get an UTI, somewhat because men's urethras are longer and progressively far off from our butts. If you're utilizing the draw out strategy, peeing between rounds of sex is going to make the probability of sperm discovering it's way to an egg uniquely more outlandish. It gets unfavorable criticism, yet the draw out technique is quite successful. (For each 100 ladies who utilize the draw out strategy consummately, 4 will get pregnant.) A part of being flawless is peeing between adjusts what will flush out left over sperm that hangs out in the urethra and diminish—however not dispense with—your odds of considering.

3Shower together.

No, showering after sex is probably not going to diminish your odds of getting a STI. What it likely will do, be that as it may, is make for an agreeable shared encounter, an approach to descend after your high and feel revived before going to bed or accomplishing something different with your day. "Sex can be untidy so if you need to shower and wash off the entirety of the liquids and sweat, put it all on the line!" says Certified Sex Therapist and Certified Sexuality Educator, Kristen Lilla, LCSW. "You could even do this together to drag out the closeness." If you have another in you, you can likewise fire things up again in the shower.

4Properly wash and set aside sex toys.

Sex toys can be marvelous and can take the delight you and your accomplice offer to an unheard of level. Things can go astray with sex toys if you don't focus on the consideration guidelines that accompany them. Research has indicated tireless organisms' capacity to stick to sex toy surfaces, so you'll be needing to clean them—yet observe the producer's suggestions, just like all different. A tissue light, for example, just requires a water wash, while butt attachments may should be bubbled. Cleanser and water may get the job done for certain items while others accompany specific cleaning liquid. "You need to try to execute the entirety of the microorganisms on them and wash off the entirety of the lube so you can take care of them," says Lilla. "Furthermore, if you clean them immediately, they'll be all set next time!" And seeing as sex toys are a fundamental piece of a couple of key situations in The 60 Sex Positions Every Couple Needs to Try, this is a measure you ought to take totally.

5Gather up utilized condoms and wrappers.

If you're utilizing condoms be a mensch and get the pre-owned ones—and remember the wrappers—and discard them appropriately: as such, don't flush them! "This is aware and exhibits that you feel similarly answerable for what you do together, " says Deborah Fox, MSW, Certified Sex Therapist. "You would prefer not to be that person who anticipates that the lady should do the housekeeping and you simply take a load off. This will deliver profits in altruism."

6Eat!

Ever seen that nourishment tastes better after you work out? For some individuals this is doubly valid for sex. A quicker hunger is only one motivation to overeat after sex, rather than previously. Feeling substantial, enlarged, and conceivably gassy after an overwhelming feast is the direct opposite of sexy. Apply a few calories, then refuel!

7Don't stop until she gets enough.

Did your accomplice have a climax during your meeting? Would she like another? If you truly need to be a sexular genius, ensure she realizes that, because sex is over for you for a brief period, that you're prepared, enthused, and ready to get her stones off with your until she taps out. "Give her you're anxious to connect more, if required" says sex advisor Constance DelGiudice, Ed.D, LMHC. "A few ladies feel they need to surge, or that they take to long. Telling her you're willing to keep with it. This will loosen up her and decrease expectant nervousness."

8Cuddle.

A typical objection among ladies that we talked with is that numerous men will turn over after sex and not have any desire to snuggle. Possibly the individual you're having intercourse with wouldn't like to nestle either yet it's a smart thought to make yourself accessible if she does. "In the wake of encountering the endorphin surge of a climax, you'll experience a discharge in oxytocin, the 'holding' substance," clarifies Lilla. "Exploit it by nestling, holding, and feeling much nearer to your accomplice."

9Emotionally interface.

Snuggling can be a piece of associating with your accomplice sincerely after sex yet there are a lot of different things you can do to keep the great vibes moving long after the headliner has reached a conclusion. You can investigate each other's eyes, synchronize your breathing, make out like young people or express your sentiments toward her. "It's particularly imperative to remain truly and genuinely present with a lady after sex," says Fox. "Ladies have made themselves defenseless against you essentially by engaging in sexual relations. Remaining associated causes her to feel sheltered and make sure about."

10Ask her what she felt about the sex you simply had.

Taking part in some focused on statistical surveying may appear to be an odd after sex action however it's as of now that her experience will be freshest in her brain and she can give you some important pointers. Reveal to her that you need and expect her genuineness and you need it so you can continue improving the sex you have together. Considering that, put your huge kid pants on and prepare to assimilate the unvarnished truth without getting guarded. Regardless of whether she reveals to you something that stings a bit, center around the possibility of a more joyful accomplice and an improved sex life.

11Address what you do and don't care for.

We as a whole have individual inclinations yet while it's anything but difficult to inform somebody that you're not insane concerning mayonnaise, it appears to be a lot trickier to be clear about your preferences in the room. All things considered, after sex is the time. "You should talk about this after sex yet not promptly subsequently in bed while that is no joke," says Lilla. "Hold up until you're both dressed, talk about it over a tidbit, in a nonpartisan setting like the kitchen, when you're not all that bare and powerless. Individuals are all the more tolerating to criticism in the correct condition." Couch your language when you're discussing stuff that you're not wild about. Rather than being negative, make statements like, "Next time, I figure it would be stunning if you... " or "I think I'd incline toward it if you slapped my can instead of tweaking my areolas."

12Compliment your accomplice.

One method for improving the sex you and your accomplice have is boosting their certainty. Studies have indicated that ladies with high confidence will in general appreciate increasingly sexual fulfillment. Except if you're a type of beast, you'll get greater delight out of sex if she's caring each moment of it. "Ladies often feel hesitant about their bodies and their appeal," says Fox. "They're besieged ordinarily every day with what the media depicts as an appealing lady, which not many can satisfy." In the radiance, disclose to her she's beautiful, that she turns you on, and how you're wild about that thing she does. Definitely, that thing.

KAMA SUTRA SEX TOP POSITIONS

Content your gathering talk about stirring up your sex life and they'll suggest it. Do a fast online inquiry and you'll be coordinated to it. Ask your mother (if that is the sort of relationship both of you have) and she'll send you a connect to arrange it on the web. That's right, I'm discussing the Kama Sutra, an old Sanskrit message that, throughout the years, has become the go-to control for multifaceted sex positions.

Because of fetishism and Western exoticism encompassing the original copy, the Kama Sutra, composed by Indian scholar Vatsyayana, has gathered a ton of consideration for its detail of what appears as though every sex position ever (some waaaay more audacious than others). Be that as it may, that is altogether not the purpose of it.

"It initially had next to no to do with sex," says Gigi Engle, a certified sex mentor. "Sex has gotten especially compared with the Kama Sutra, however, it's a profound book." truth be told, the guide is tied in with supporting connections—with just one segment committed to genuine positions.

All things considered, the segment is a powerful one. It's stuffed with A TON of sex places that advance passionate closeness between accomplices by method for contact and physical association. The old content even trains that men ought to organize a lady's pleasure over their own (hear!), by concentrating on ensuring she peaks before considering their own climax.

And keeping in mind that the following level positions are interesting, Engle wouldn't prescribe the greater part of them...unless you are excessively dexterous and physically slanted. The ones that merit concentrating on (if you consider yourself as a real part of us unflexibles), she says, are the easier moves that don't include insane backbends or put you in danger of pulling a hammy.

"It's less about going in and having the option to do these different positions; it's progressively about discovering ones that you can adjust," Engle says. It's increasingly significant that you come into the night (or morning, or restroom fast in and out) with energy, as "that is the thing that separates great sex from incredible sex," she guarantees. By the day's end, experimentation is tied in with being available with your accomplice and indicating each other that you're willing to do as well as you possibly can.

Since you realize that...ready to give these 10 Kama Sutra sex positions a spin?

1 The Om

Called Padmasana or Lotus in the first Kama Sutra message, this energetic position is one that, as per Engle, is best done by pounding against your accomplice for clitoral incitement, instead of ricocheting here and there. If you're on your accomplice you can bring down yourself onto their penis or a dildo, or if entrance's not your thing, you can rub facing them for outercourse.

Do It: Your accomplice sits leg over leg (yoga-/pretzel-style); you sit in their lap confronting them. Fold your legs over them and embrace each other for help.

2 G-Whiz

This is a decent decision if you and your accomplice aren't particularly adaptable, since the move just necessitates that you can twist at the abdomen. Furthermore, "if you have a tallness difference, you can put a few cushions underneath the other individual, or you can use a sex pad," says Engle.

Do It: With your accomplice sitting on their knees, lie back with your legs laying on every one of your accomplice's shoulders.

3 Enchantment Mountain

While this scissoring-type move fits infiltration, it's likewise an incredible one for young lady on-young lady sex, where accomplices can physically animate each other with either a toy or their hands.

Do It: Your accomplice sits, legs bowed, reclining on all fours. You do likewise, and afterward crawl toward them until you reach.

4 The Chairman

This is another sex position where you may think bobbing is the correct move, at the same time, once more, crushing is certainly the best approach. The Chairman is an extraordinary starter move for profound infiltration, having your accomplice kiss your shoulders and your neck, and for areola play, as well.

Do you want to take things up a score? Get a sex toy and have your accomplice stretch around you for manual incitement.

Do It: Your accomplice sits on the edge of the bed and you sit on them, confronting endlessly.

5 Preacher

"Preacher is one of the most underestimated positions," says Engle. Indeed, as "fundamental" all things considered, it's a Kama Sutra sex position: "There are such a large number of different varieties," and it's v personal (all that nearby eye to eye connection = all the feels).

Have a go at stacking pads underneath your pelvis with the goal that your accomplice on top can push in an upward corner to corner heading, granulating against your clitoris.

Do It: Lie on your back while your accomplice lies facedown on you.

6 The Pinball Wizard

This is a primo Kama Sutra move for profound entrance, says Engle. In any case, if you can't hold a scaffold position, or your accomplice can't bolster your lower body with their arms, perhaps proceed onward to something different (because over-effort isn't sexy).

Do It: You get into an incomplete extension position (like a pinball machine), with your weight laying on your shoulders. Your accomplice enters you from a bowing position.

7 Switch Cowgirl

This present one's somewhat more of a test, says Engle, since the common bend of most penises or tie ons don't generally oblige this position, however it's feasible. (No big surprise ladies will in general abhor on this sex position.) Once you get your depression, it's a decent time.

Master tip: To up your scope of development when you're on top, Engle proposes putting a cushion under every knee.

Do It: Your accomplice lies on their back; you straddle them, confronting their feet.

8 Stand and Deliver

If you're feeling particularly bold, attempt the Stand and Deliver. It's a Kama Sutra–endorsed move that is useful for shallow entrance in its present condition. If you're searching for more profound infiltration, you can bring it down to your knees rather—an adjustment which, Engle says, is an incredible method to make up for a tallness difference.

What's more, if you're the individual on the less than desirable end and you're stressed over falling when things get sweat-soaked, Engle says to incline toward a table or a seat for help.

Do It: With both of you standing, you twist around at the midriff; they enter you from behind.

9 Ballet artist

If balance begins to get extreme while you and your accomplice are grinding away right now, don't get baffled, says Engle. Rather, turn. "Drop to your knees, and you can give that individual a penis massage or cunnilingus, or the other way around." interestingly, you gave it a go.

Do It: Standing on one foot, face your accomplice and fold your other leg over their abdomen while they help bolster you.

10 The Good Ex

This close position is simpler than it looks, says Engle. "It's an incredible chance to acquire something like a wand vibrator" for you to use on yourself simultaneously. What's more, whoever is in the situated position, shaking to and fro, may likewise consider utilizing a butt plug for included incitement.

Do It: Sit on the bed confronting each other with legs forward. Lift your accomplice's correct leg over your left and lift your correct leg over their left. Meet up so they can enter you. Presently, both of you lie back, your legs framing a X. Slow, lackadaisical gyrations supplant pushing. Hi, closeness!

A couple thousand years back, when Indian author Vatsyayana was putting pen to paper and composing the content that would be known as the Kama Sutra, he was unable to have anticipated the effect that his work would have on the world. In the cutting edge period, the words "Kama Sutra" are an equivalent word for sex. Various outlets have utilized "Kama Sutra" to signify "insane approaches to do it," from the (sincere) Cosmo Kama Sutra to the (profoundly unapproved) spoof Star Wars Kama Sutra; go to kamasutra.com and you'll discover an organization represent considerable authority in "extravagance sentiment and closeness items," like palatable body paints and cleans.

If it appears to be unusual that a 2,000-year-old content keeps on conveying such effect on our sexual minds, it gets significantly more peculiar when you understand that a large portion of the Kama Sutra isn't in reality about sex. Not at all like the numerous hot-and-overwhelming sex manuals that bear its name, the first Kama Sutra is philosophical content contribution thoughts on the best way to have a compensating life and productive connections; to the degree that it's a sex manual, it's for the most part because it doesn't avoid the idea that sex (and fascinating sex positions) is a solid and typical piece of life. (Obviously, given this is a 2,000-year-old content, it's exceptionally heteronormative — while strange sex and non-regularizing sex characters do show up in the content, the general supposition that will be that the peruser's essential sexual relationship will be a heterosexual one.)

Be that as it may, some place down the line (and most likely because of quite orientalism), the non-sex portions of the Kama Sutra got overlooked, and the sex parts got developed — and, now and again, completely rethought (stunning as it might appear, Vatsyayana didn't expound on sex acts including separable shower heads).

So what's very the first Kama Sutra? A wide assortment of stuff – including, indeed, loads of sex positions. How about we investigate the sex positions supported by the old tome.

As per the Kamasutra, there are 64 kinds of sexual acts one can take a stab at during lovemaking. They change, obviously, from being perplexing muscle developments to delicate, sexy stances. Have you at any point needed to attempt every one of them, and pondered, simultaneously, if there would one say one is implied exceptionally for you?

In fact talking, sex is an odd impossible to miss thing: we have two individuals sitting in places that appear to oppose the gravitational laws, puffing and moving quickly while they are trading liquids. Sex can, indeed, become exhausting and disagreeable as it similarly is fulfilling and valuable.

The more imaginative you are and the more you attempt to make a wonderful climate in bed, the better you will feel, because you will have the option to convey positive emotions to your accomplice. If you consider as a real part of the individuals who engage in sexual relations for delight and if everything happens normally and gratitude to your body life systems, bravo! However, if you or her have certain weight issues and you can't generally bear to attempt any wild stuff in bed, here are a portion of your choices for different sorts of outlines...

Doggy style

If you are both going up against some undesirable kilos, you can attempt the accompanying: she lays on her back and effectively twists her knees, and you remain between her legs and raise them during entrance. Another reasonable situation for you is the doggy style, which all in all is a charming one for the two accomplices.

Butterfly position

If you have an ideal weight, and your accomplice is well proportioned, she will remain on a side, while you raise her leg to the chest level or as much as her adaptability permits her to. Then tenderly slide towards her and hold her leg while entering her. Additionally, you can remain before your accomplice, whose legs dangle over the edge of a bed or some other stage like a table; with your accomplice's legs lifted towards the roof and leaning against you, this is here and there called the "butterfly position". It should likewise be possible as a stooping position.

Switched Cowgirl position

If she has the ideal weight, and you are overweight, sit on your back, while she remains above you with her face situated towards your legs. Curve your knees, while she moves remaining on your knees. This position is known as the "turned around cowgirl".

Spoon position

If you are altogether different as far as stature, the "spoon position" is the perfect one for you. You both need to sit on a side, with you being behind her. You will appreciate some fairly cool moves as this position is incredibly private, wonderful and appropriate to anyone type.

Janakurpara position

If you and your accomplice have fit bodies, then Janukurpara position is only for you. It requires both of you to have solid abs, and you may wind up consuming a great deal of calories. Start with lifting her up and bolting your elbows under her knees to improve hold. Hold her butt with your hands and let her hold you from your neck.

This position offers additional profound infiltration, and therefore loads of joy. Also, it prompts a great deal of eye to eye connection that adds to the experience. Janakurpara position is the award for all the difficult exercise you have done in the rec center to get the fit body.

Tripadam position

This sex position works best when both the accomplices are of same tallness, but on the other hand it's an extraordinary attempt when you are in a state of mind of a quick in and out, Tripadam position can end up being stunning for you-it's short, quick and you needn't bother with a bed for it.

Right now, both stand confronting one another. You lift one of her knees and spot your hand under it. This position is alluded as Tripadam or tripod, and doesn't permit profound infiltration.

Like the various standing positions, this position likewise elevates greatest blood stream to your erogenous zones, and ensures you make some great memories.

Piditaka position

Piditaka is agreeable, laid-back position and should be possible by anybody, whenever of the day! Let her twist her knees and spot on your chest. In the meantime, place your knees on the either side of her rump, and lift her thighs a smidgen, and enter her.

This sex position ensures delight as the vagina is limited when the legs are up. Besides, you can pass on quietude, love and delicacy by letting her legs contact your mouth and feet.

By the by, the most significant thing you and your accomplice should remember is that there are no severe standards in bed; you should offer yourself to your accomplice and get her fondness however you see fit, your creative mind go out of control. There is no comparative inclination to that of giving and similarly getting delight from the individual you love.

FLEXIBILITY POSITIONS

We're continually hearing that we could be having better sex, a superior climax, or a superior relationship. Be that as it may, how often do we hear the quick and dirty of how we can in reality better comprehend our most profound wants and most humiliating inquiries? Clamor has enrolled Vanessa Marin, a sex advisor, to assist us with excursion with the subtleties. No sex, sexual direction, or question is beyond reach, and all inquiries stay mysterious. Presently, onto the present point: the best sex positions for adaptable and tough individuals.

Q: I'm laying down with a person I met in yoga class, and allows simply state we've been having a fabulous time getting progressively adaptable together! What are some enjoyment, unordinary sex positions we could attempt? He's really solid as well, and I need to exploit it.

A: Thanks for the inquiry! Evaluating new positions is one of the best time parts of sex, and being adaptable surely opens up an entirely different universe of potential outcomes. Here are seven extraordinary situations for individuals who have been investing some additional energy at the rec center. (Note: these positions have been portrayed and depicted here utilizing a man and a lady, yet two ladies could surely appreciate these positions utilizing a tie on.)

1. The Ankle Choker

The most effective method to do it: Start off in Missionary. Prop up your knees so your feet are laying on the bed. Have your person gradually begin to sit up and raise up on his knees. Raise your hips up into connect present so he remains within you. He can likewise help by hanging on under your hips. Gradually raise one advantage and lay it on his shoulder, then rehash with your other leg. Contingent upon your stature differences, you can inch your lower legs further up his shoulders, or he can utilize his hands to raise your pelvis up higher. From that point, you hold tight for the ride while he pushes all through you.

Why it's enjoyment: This is an incredible situation for hitting your G-spot. Having your legs together will make an enticingly full inclination. You can crush a hand between your thighs for some extra clitoral incitement. You'll be on the whole topsy turvy, which is entirely novel. Furthermore, you'll get a pleasant hamstring and calf stretch all the while!

2. The Advanced Crab Walk

Step by step instructions to do it: Have him plunk down with his arms propped behind him. Gradually lower yourself onto him, straddling his hips. Recline with the goal that your weight is laying on your hands. Each in turn, test your sanity up to lay on his shoulders. You can't push that much, so you'll need to concentrate more on shaking or pounding against one another. You can utilize your lower legs for some additional influence.

Why it's enjoyment: This position is a decent moderate burner since there's a constrained scope of development. Having your legs near one another can make for a pleasant tight fit. Both of you will get an overly hot perspective on him sliding all through you.

3. The Seated Backbend

The most effective method to do it: Have him sit up. Lower yourself onto him, putting one knee on either side of his body. Gradually begin to lean in reverse into a backbend. You can have him hold your hips to manage your development. You can lay on your upper back, or prop yourself up on your lower arms. Concentrate on shaking against one another, or pounding your hips in moderate circles. Possibly you or he can reach down and rub your clitoris.

Why it's enjoyment: This is another position that is a decent, slow bother. It can likewise be very private, since he can contact all over your body. He can give specific consideration to your clitoris, since it will be up front for him.

4. The Bouncing Reverse Cowgirl

Step by step instructions to do it: Have him set down on the finish of the bed, with his legs hung over the edge and feet level on the ground. Remain between his legs, confronting a similar course as he may be. Lower yourself onto him. You're in finished control during this position. You can sway here and there on his penis, or pound around and around.

Why it's enjoyment: This is an adaptable position. You can sit in the middle of his legs, or put your legs outside of his. You can lean advances or in reverse to change the point of infiltration. Having your feet level on the ground gives you substantially more influence and control than the typical lady on-top positions where you're on your knees. You can without much of a stretch stroke your clitoris, and he can undoubtedly animate your rear-end.

5. The Splitter

Step by step instructions to do it: Lie on your side, and raise one leg into the air. Have him straddle the leg that is lying on the bed and hurry forward until he enters you. You can rest the leg that is noticeable all around on his shoulder, or he can clutch it for influence. He pushes all through you.

Why it's enjoyment: This is an extremely sexy position that will cause you to feel thankful for all that yoga parts practice! This position can make exceptionally profound, extreme incitement. Both of you can give your clitoris some additional incitement.

6. The Plow

The most effective method to do it: Start off in Missionary. Have him sit up for a minute so you can test your sanity back out of sight and lay your shoulders on his lower legs. He can gradually bring down himself towards you. How far he can go relies upon your adaptability. When you're into position, he pushes as he ordinarily would in Missionary.

Why it's enjoyment: This is a ground-breaking, bestial situation with extremely profound infiltration. You'll feel completely overwhelmed by him.

7. Standing Rear-Entry

Instructions to do it: Have him remain behind you. Spread your legs and twist around a piece to make it simpler for him to enter you. When he's inside, unite your legs and twist around as far as possible. Check whether you can get your hands level on the ground (or on a yoga obstruct) for some additional influence. He can hold your hips for influence as he pushes all through you. This one works best for couples that don't have a lot of stature difference, however you can utilize a stool or a stair to make it work.

Why it's enjoyment: Any back passage position is incredible for G-spot incitement. The way that he's standing will give him extraordinary influence for extreme, incredible pushing. Having your legs near one another will make an excessively tight fit. This is another position where you'll get a decent stretch!

SIXTH BOOK: Kama Sutra for Beginners and Sex Positions

INTRODUCTION OF KAMA SUTRA

The Kama Sutra is an old Indian Sanskrit message on sexuality, suggestion and passionate satisfaction in life. Ascribed to Vātsyāyana, the Kama Sutra is neither solely nor transcendently a sex manual on sex positions, however composed as a manual for the "craft of-living" great, the nature of adoration, finding a life accomplice, keeping up one's affection life, and different viewpoints relating to joy situated resources of human life.

Kamasutra is the most seasoned enduring Hindu content on sensual love. It is a sutra-kind content with pithy aphoristic stanzas that have made due into the cutting edge time with different bhasya (composition and editorials). The content is a blend of composition and anustubh-meter verse sections. The content recognizes the Hindu idea of Purusharthas, and records want, sexuality, and passionate satisfaction as one of the best possible objectives of life. Its sections talk about strategies for romance, preparing in expressions of the human experience to be socially captivating, finding an accomplice, being a tease, keeping up power in a wedded life, when and how to submit infidelity, sexual positions, and different themes. Most of the book is about the way of thinking and hypothesis of affection, what triggers want, what supports it, and how and when it is positive or negative.

The content is one of numerous Indian messages on Kama Shastra. It is a much-interpreted work in Indian and non-Indian dialects. The Kamasutra has impacted numerous optional writings that trailed the fourth century CE, just as the Indian expressions as exemplified by the inescapable nearness Kama-related reliefs and figure in old Hindu sanctuaries. Of these, the Khajuraho in Madhya Pradesh is an UNESCO world legacy site. Among the enduring sanctuaries in north India, one in Rajasthan shapes all the significant parts and sexual positions to represent the Kamasutra.

As indicated by Wendy Doniger, the Kamasutra became "one of the most pilfered books in English language" not long after it was distributed in 1883 by Richard Burton. This first European version by Burton doesn't reliably reflect much in the Kamasutra because he overhauled the shared interpretation by Bhagavanlal Indrajit and Shivaram Parashuram Bhide with Forster Arbuthnot to suit nineteenth century Victorian tastes.

HISTORY AND PHILOSOPHY OF KAMA SUTRA

The first creation date or century for the Kamasutra is obscure. History specialists have differently put it between 400 BCE and 300 CE. According to John Keay, the Kama Sutra is an abridgment that was gathered into its present structure in the second century CE. interestingly, the Indologist Wendy Doniger who has co-interpreted Kama sutra and distributed numerous papers on related Hindu messages, the enduring form of the Kamasutra more likely than not been reconsidered or created after 225 CE because it makes reference to the Abhiras and the Andhras lines that didn't co-rule significant districts of old India before that year. The content makes no notice of the Gupta Empire which governed over major urban regions of old India, reshaping antiquated Indian expressions, Hindu culture and economy from the fourth century through the sixth century. Therefore, she dates the Kama sutra to the second 50% of the third century CE.

The spot of its piece is additionally hazy. The imaginable applicants are urban focuses of north or northwest antiquated India, on the other hand in the eastern urban Pataliputra (presently Patna).

Vatsyayana Mallanaga is its generally acknowledged creator because his name is implanted in the colophon section, yet little is thought about him. Vatsyayana states that he composed the content after much meditation. In the introduction, Vatsyayana recognizes that he is refining numerous antiquated writings, yet these have not survived. He refers to crafted by others he calls "instructors" and "researchers", and the more drawn out writings by Auddalaki, Babhravya, Dattaka, Suvarnanabha, Ghotakamukha, Gonardiya, Gonikaputra, Charayana, and Kuchumara. Vatsyayana's Kamasutra is referenced and a few stanzas cited in the Brihatsamhita of Varahamihira, just as the sonnets of Kalidasa. This recommends he lived before the fifth century CE.

Regardless of whether you would prefer not to let it be known, I thoroughly consider many individuals there would truly value having a Guide to Sex – - actually no, not your secondary school sex-ed instructor ungracefully staying a condom on a banana, or late-night, incorrectly spelled Google look on in secret mode–a complete, bit by bit manual for affection, sex, enthusiasm and everything in the middle. Wouldn't that be pleasant?

All things considered, I have news for you. It exists! Also, it's really been around longer than you might suspect. A LOT longer.

The "Kama Sutra" (here and there showed as single word, "Kamasutra") is accepted to be expounded in on ADE 320 to 550 India (during the Gupta

Golden Age) by a strict understudy and logician named Vatsyayana. The title makes an interpretation of generally to "The Aphorism of Desire," or "The Formula of Lust," contingent upon who you inquire.

A great many people know it as the insidious book you found in your flower child auntie's home, and that it's predominantly involved a rundown of preposterously athletic-looking sexual positions. Nothing could be more distant from reality.

Above all else, the book is situated in Hinduism, which implies that it's in fact a strict book. In Hinduism there are four fundamentals, or objectives, of human life that all individuals must accomplish;

Dharma (Duty and ethicalness),

Artha (reason and embodiment),

Kama (Desire and energy) and

Moksha (self-realization).

The Kamasutra was basically a manual for accomplishing the "want" objective of these precepts.

Just around 20 percent of the book – one section, to be accurate arrangements with the subject of sexual positions. The remainder of the books manage the subjects of want, desire, enchantment and the way of thinking of affection.

Presently, remember that in old India, sex and sexuality was a huge piece of Indian culture. Polygamy and polyamory were normal, particularly in the high societies. Nakedness in craftsmanship was plentiful, and sex was viewed as a conjugal obligation for the wife, yet for the spouse as well. In spite of the fact that it was an exclusive arrangement, the two accomplices were relied upon to delight each other in the demonstration.

The Kama Sutra is for the most part written in exposition in the stanza structure, isolated into 36, here and there 35, sections and seven sections. The primary segment, isolated into four sections, goes over affection when all is said in done, alongside the job of "delegates," or partners, to aid the securing of a sweetheart and life objectives.

The subsequent part is the most notable, and contains 10 sections on sexual positions, sexual methods, for example, oral sex and butt-centric, gnawing, groaning, slapping and foreplay.

The third and fourth segments are seven sections altogether, enumerating the complexities of acquiring a wife, marriage, wifely obligations and the consideration and treatment of a wife. The fifth section, all things considered, talks about the strategies of enticing others' spouses.

The 6th segment has six sections that go over concubines, or escorts, the securing of such and companions with benefits. The seventh and last segment remembers two sections for drawing in individuals and utilizing sexual ability to improve physical fascination.

The Kama sutra was first interpreted and distributed in 1883 by Indian prehistorian Bhagwan Lal Indraji, and has since been reproduced on various occasions. More up to date interpretations started to spring up in the 60's and 70's during the sexual upset, and in the 90's the most enticing piece of the book, the 64 sexual positions, began to make their rounds on the early gatherings of the Internet. Along these lines, a great many people feel this is the main segment of the book.

If you get an opportunity, get the Kama Sutra. It's somewhat ancient regarding sexual orientation fairness, yet it has a few pieces of intelligence to a great extent. Furthermore, recall: Always stretch before you work out, and if it looks excruciating give it a pass.

NEW DELHI — Yoga is hard for most Indians, as well, and they positively don't rehearse it while engaging in sexual relations. They likely never endeavored such a mix in their entire history. The worldwide view that old Indians performed outrageous acrobatic while having intercourse was seeded by a late-nineteenth century English interpretation of a Sanskrit content called the Kama Sutra, which contained, in addition to other things, subtleties of sexual positions, pragmatic counsel on enchantment and a note on sorts of suggestive ladies, who were named after warm blooded creatures despite the fact that, as a book discharged for the current month watches, they made commotions like flying creatures.

"The Mare's Trap: Nature and Culture in the Kamasutra" by Wendy Doniger, an American scholarly, contends, as some perceiving couples may have suspected, that the sex in the Kama Sutra is more trick than instructional manual. In any case, the stupendous desire of her book is to raise the Kama Sutra to the status of two incredible philosophical works that have affected Indian culture: Manu's Dharmashastra, which designed positions and characterized ladies as subordinate to men, humiliating some fine individuals who share the writer's name, and Kautilya's Arthashastra, a merciless book on statecraft.

Next to no is thought about the roots of the Kama Sutra. No segment of the first content has endure. It was likely written in Sanskrit by one Vatsyayana. He appears to have been a compiler of sexual propensities, and he reprimanded another researcher for concocting a portion of the difficult sexual positions. Ms. Doniger accepts that the Kama Sutra is around 2,000 years of age, yet she revealed to me this depends exclusively on conditional proof.

The explanation she pays attention to the Kama Sutra so is that despite the fact that she feels that the sexual positions were dreams, she finds in the remainder of the work out and out human sciences, an uncommon representation of a wealthy old society. Additionally, there are elaborate similitudes between the Kama Sutra and crafted by Manu and Kautilya. Every one of the three incorporate mental investigations and guidelines and separation individuals into types.

The Kama Sutra is for and about the rich. It has next to no to say about the poor aside from as sexual prey. Ms. Doniger suspects it was initially a seven-demonstration play about the craft of adoration. The anonymous hero is alluded to as nagaraka, a "man-about-town." He is urban and rich. He has "a froth shower each third day," the Kama Sutra says, "his body hair expelled each fifth or tenth day ... and he persistently cleans the perspiration from his armpits."

Similarly as with men today, his penis is libertarian. This is a significant disclosure of the Kama Sutra, as per Ms. Doniger, because it appears to resist the laws of Manu that isolate society into ranks and denounces their blending.

The Kama Sutra doesn't preclude ladies, either, from having flings with those in the lower positions, however it asks them to be reasonable. It seems to depict a general public that was far less inflexible than what Manu appointed, and that was more amicable to ladies.

Manu says, "Great looks don't make a difference to them [women], nor do they care about youth. 'A man!' they state and appreciate sex with him." But Vatsyayana says a lady wants "any appealing man" similarly as "a man wants a lady. Be that as it may, after some thought [by the woman], the issue goes no further."

While Manu needs to control ladies, Vatsyayana underestimates female wantonness. He says that men who need to get hitched ladies would have a decent possibility in sanctuaries, at weddings and, for reasons unknown, in the region of a house that is ablaze.

BENEFITS OF THE KAMA SUTRA

In the West, "Kama Sutra" is by all accounts synonymous with flexibility specialist sex positions – ones that join trapeze artistry, yoga, and maybe antiquated sex entertainment.

All things considered, this is just halfway evident.

All things considered, the Kama Sutra covers significantly more than meets the Western eye, and to consider the Kama Sutra a book of hot sex positions is doing this sacrosanct, old Hindu content a tremendous damage.

Here's the reason,

It's not extravagant positions that transform regular sex into tantric, sacrosanct, lovemaking – that is just extremely about 20% of it. Genuine, consecrated lovemaking is for the most part about soul and association, which is absolutely why the sexual positions just make up about 20% of the Kama Sutra.

The remainder of this hallowed content is a guide on the Art of Love and Living Virtuously; including, yet surely not restricted to:

The way of thinking and nature of adoration

Family life

What triggers want (and what continues it)

Decorum

Self-care

Appropriate preparing

The act of different expressions, for example, scent blending, verse, and cooking

Adjusting female and manly energies (in oneself and inside an association)

Numerous different resources of (non-sexual) joy arranged features of life

kamasutra

What Is Kamasutra?

Things being what they are, precisely what is Kamasutra?

"Kamasutra" originates from two different Sanskrit words – "kama" and "sutra". Each word has an unequivocal importance. Joined, the two implications make up the reason of the book.

The historical background of Kama Sutra: The most exciting approach to analyze words to assemble meaning!

Kama

"Kama" in Sanskrit implies want and is comprised of both sexy and stylish wants. In any case, as to the Kamasutra, an accentuation is put on sexy want.

The word kama is the Sanskrit can signify "love," "want," or "delight." This joy isn't restricted to sexual want, but instead an expansive term enveloping all the joys of life.

In most world religions, sexual want is viewed as unthinkable.

Be that as it may, Hinduism holds "kama" as one of the Four Goals of Hindu Life. In their objectives of life, "kama" is trailed by "artha" (plenitude, achievement), "dharma" (prudence, truth), and "moksha" (discharge).

Sutra

"Sutra" in Sanskrit implies line or string. It is a similar root as the English word suture, the strands of a line that are utilized in medication to seal wounds. In any case, Sutra here alludes to the alludes to a string of sections that structure a manual.

kama

Where Does The Kama Sutra Come From?

The Kama Sutra was a book composed between 400 – 200 BCE. The Indian logician and sage who composed it, Vātsyāyana Mallanaga, incorporated sexual lessons and astuteness as a type of contemplation.

He professed to be a chaste priest and didn't record these lessons from individual experience. Or maybe, he dense the exercises from the Kamashastra (the Rules of Love), which was made hundreds out of years sooner.

Investigating The Kama Sutra Book

The Kamasutra was written in an extract and darken type of Sanskrit. Portions of it remain very tricky and unrelatable in our cutting edge period, in any event, when meant English.

Refering to crafted by different creators and sutras of a lot more seasoned writings, Vātsyāyana arranged what we are aware of today as the Kama Sutra. It was written in a fairly intricate and theoretical type of Sanskrit. It has 1,250 sections that are part into 36 parts and further sorted out into 7 different parts.

Kama Sutra book

The Kama Sutra book is separated into 7 sections

1. Dattaka – General standards

The initial segment is a presentation and foundation of the 4 points of Hindu life, the Kama specifically. It introduces the whole book with bits of shrewdness and theory on subjects, for example, how to secure information and how to live decently.

2. Suvarnanabha – Amorous advances and sexual association

The subsequent part makes a plunge directly into the antiquated explicit thoughts numerous westerners partner with the Kamasutra. It subtleties 64 different sorts of sexual acts, for example, grasping, kissing, groaning, slapping, sexual positions, and different types of erotica.

3. Ghotakamukha – Acquiring a wife

The third segment manages living as a lone ranger and strategies for pursuing a lady for marriage. These techniques aren't exactly fitting for current occasions and are for the most part dependent on mysterious similarity and the advantages of marriage for the families in question (station frameworks).

4. Gonardiya – Duties, and benefits of the wife

This segment talks about the obligations of the wife: cooking, cleaning, and taking into account the spouse. While these uneven sex jobs may have appeared well and good 3,000 years prior, they are not all that fitting for present-day connections.

5. Gonikaputra – Other men's spouses

The fifth part depicts the jobs of guys and females in a relationship with respect to non-sexual closeness. It incorporates understanding passionate estimations and talks about approaches to extend enthusiastic securities.

6. Charayana – Courtesans

The focal point of this segment is the man's utilization of mistresses, or whores, to fabricate certainty before seeking after a wife. It likewise offers guidance on repairing past associations with companions and darlings, accomplishing riches, and finding a submitted accomplice.

7. Kuchumara – Occult practices

The Kama Sutra completes with an area on sexual fantasies, legends, and practices to keep things energizing. This incorporates individual prepping, the utilization of scents and oils, home solutions for sexual brokenness, and that's only the tip of the iceberg.

Here is an extract from the Kamasutra with respect to the assortments of groaning during sex:

"The whine, the moan, the jibber jabber, the howl, the murmur, the yell, the cry and words with significance, for example, 'Mother!' 'Stop!' 'Let go!' or 'Enough!' Cries like those of birds, cuckoos, green pigeons, parrots, honey bees, moorhens, geese, ducks, and quails are significant choices for use in groaning."

... Not exactly your 21st-century sonic scene.

Fortunately, there has since been a refreshed rendition of the Kamasutra. The fifteenth century gave us the Ananga-Ranga, a considerably more brief and fathomable content about human sexual delight, which, for a long time, really supplanted the Kama Sutra.

Inside and out, the Kamasutra can be seen as a manual for temperate living, investigating the nature and reasoning of affection, develops of family life, and the different parts of joy and want.

A great many people believe that learning is simply the key advancement.

It's the means by which we were raised – when we were youthful, we contemplated variable based math, read history, and retained the names of components on the occasional table.

In any case, when you grow up and experience life, you understand that you can't 'learn' certain things – like self-awareness.

Vishen Lakhiani, organizer of Mindvalley and New York Times Bestselling creator, found that the way to self-advancement was not to 'learn', but instead, to 'change'.

INTERMEDIATE SEX POSITIONS OF KAMA SUTRA

Tingling for some new and imaginative sex positions? Regardless of whether you have an inclination that you've just taken a stab at everything in the book, you'll locate some hot AF proceeds onward this rundown sure to astonish you. We have a wide range of sex positions to take a stab at this ace rundown, with moves from the Kama Sutra to current perfect works of art roused by Kim and Kanye (you heard us right).

Try not to misunderstand us: There's a great deal to be said for the old reserve moves like teacher and cowgirl—also the unlimited minor departure from them. In any case, if you're searching for all the more a test, these inventive sex positions have you secured. In addition, none of these positions are unusual to the point that pitching them to your accomplice will be ungainly. Win-win.

So continue perusing and find innovative sex positions that will offer have even the most unquenchable perusers of sex tips taking notes.

1. The Bouncy Chair

In the first place, guide him to get down on his knees (this is fun, as of now!). Have him bow with his butt behind him and the bundles of his feet on the ground. Straddle his lap, confronting him with you feet level on the floor on either side of his legs. When you're in position (and his erect penis is inside you), ricochet on the chunks of your feet to control the musicality and infiltration. The nearness will make for some delightful private time and you'll get the discharge you so urgently need.

2. Lotus

Straight out of the Kama Sutra, the Lotus position is a blast from the past that is certain to flavor things up. In spite of the fact that it requires a touch of adaptability, the result is absolutely justified, despite all the trouble. Here's the means by which it goes: Lie on your back and fold your legs "Indian style." Now, bring your legs (despite everything crossed) as carefully shrouded as could be allowed and have your man jump on top. Keep up the leg over leg position as long as you can hack it. It's a major hip opener, yet the perfect plot for a g-spot climax.

3. Parting the Bamboo

You know how some of the time following a monotonous day, the exact opposite thing you need to do is lash on your chaps and ride your way around the room? All things considered, relax, cowgirls, this Kama Sutra sex position is your companion. Start by lying on your back and have your man accept minister position. Then raise one leg and lay it on his shoulder up by his head.

Keep the other leg loosened up on the bed. You'll see that with one leg noticeable all around, entrance will feel much more profound. If you're awkward or your hamstrings are not as adaptable as you'd trusted, request that he stoop. In any case, if he's still watching out for that g-spot of yours, "Parting of a Bamboo" will improve his chances of discovering it.

4. Milk and Water

Discover a seat (ideally one without arms) and cause him to sit his bare self down. Then sit down on his lap, confronting endlessly from him, and lead his hand to any place it is you like to be contacted. When you can't take the prodding any longer, re-position yourself with the goal that he's within you while you're despite everything sitting on him. Urge him to continue contacting you while you move to and fro until either of you peak. Sounds incredibly hot, isn't that right?

5. Generally Opened

Falsehood level on your back. Have your man stoop on the bed with his knees marginally separated, and fold your legs over his abdomen. Then raise your hips and pelvis by angling your back and flaunting your heavenly boobs. Have him bolster you at the little of your back while he does the pushing. That is everything to "Generally Opened." Really, is there anything sexier than a lady curving her back?

6. Tigress

Think switch cowgirl with a contort. Have your man rests and sit on him, confronting endlessly. Presently reach back and place one hand on his masculine chest. Utilize your hand to stable yourself as you go all over. This permits you to have unlimited authority over the speed and profundity of entrance. You can likewise have him put his hands on your abdomen if you discover you need a lift. The additional in addition to? You'll have the option to glance back at him taking a gander at you, which will undoubtedly help things along.

7. The Pretzel

You lay on your side with your base leg under him and the other folded over his stomach. As far as concerns him, he ought to stoop down. This position augments the potential for profound, fulfilling pushes, and the sideways edge truly shakes things up for new and energizing sensations.

8. Standing Wheel Barrow

This one will truly get the blood racing to your head, and is a simple accomplishment for committed yogis. Expect descending pooch position and afterward let your accomplice tenderly get your legs and fold them over his midsection. You'll bolster yourself with your arms and for included help, he'll likewise hold you by your hips as he the light in him praises the light in you. Namaste.

9. Cascade

This is a contort on the great young lady on top we as a whole know and love. This adaptation, in any case, leaves you absolutely in charge. He should set down on the bed, however then hurry in reverse so his chest area is hung on the bed and onto the floor at edge. When he's set, straddle him and ride him as he appreciates the view from underneath.

10. Wellness Friends

Astroglide's occupant sexologist "Dr. Jess" O'Reilly, Ph.D., gave this position its name because it would appear that you're doing a helped leg lift. You lie on your side with one advantage, and your accomplice sits on their knees, straddles your base leg, and enters you while adjusting your lower leg on their shoulder.

11. The Spider

Recall doing the crab stroll in exercise center class (or possibly more as of late at an innovative Crossfit meeting)? The two accomplices get into crab strolling position and compromise. Both the your legs ought to be inside his legs are outside. Since you're on top, lift up your pelvis to bring down yourself on your accomplice. From that point, you control the shaking. It's designated "The Spider" because this one looks practically like the name would propose.

12. Standing 69

Dr. Jess prescribes this to stir up the exemplary common oral sex position. One individual stands upstanding, and the different goes into a handstand while different holds them. This ought to permit you both to arrive at one another's insidious bits, however you may need to stop it before all the blood races to your head. This may be all the more a "fair to state we did it" sort of position, truly.

13. X Marks the Spot

For this turn on evangelist, put your advantages and either keep them straight or lay your feet on your accomplice's chest. That is when the "X" part comes in: Cross your legs to make a more tightly fit for more contact.

14. Devious Tee

To handle another piece of the letters in order, lie on your back with your feet level and your legs twisted, then have your accomplice slide beneath your legs so you structure a T shape, thus the name (another Dr. Jess coinage).

15. Standing Tiger Crouching Dragon

Doin' it from behind gets a ton more blazing with this straightforward variety. Bow on the bed (or sofa or eating table or floor or any raised surface) let him enter you from behind. This permits him to hit different points than if you were simply twisted around. Star tip: The sensation will changed dependent on how far separated you place your legs. Play with opening your legs more extensive and smaller to discover what feels best to you.

16. Stunt-devils

If you're hoping to get a pleasant stretch in to your next sex meeting, have we got the situation for you. Lie on your back with your legs over your head and your butt up as though you were doing a regressive roll, and have your accomplice enter you from the side. Hello, it hasn't called Acrobats to no end.

17. The Bound 2

Picture may contain Human Person Hand and Hug

Commercial

We don't need you to really ride a cruiser while you engage in sexual relations (that would be perilous!). Rather, utilize some of Kim Kardashian and Kanye West's preferred embellishments: a mirror, your telephone (for taking selfies mid-lovemaking, obviously), and arranged shopping packs from Givenchy and Balmain strewn about the space to set the state of mind. Your man sits on a position of authority (or a seat, if you don't have a royal position convenient), confronting a mirror. You roost on his lap, taking looks at the mirror. No real sex is required; you simply get off on how hot you look.

18. The Hashtag

It is a pound sign all things considered (get it?). To take on the position: Lie on your side while your person stoops confronting you and lifts up your top leg (like the scissors position).

19. The iPhone X

Propelled by Apple's energizing new dispatch, this move praises that greater is better. Lie on your back and push your hips up into an extension (keep your head and neck on the floor while supporting yourself with your shoulders).

Your person remains on the bed straddling you, holding your hips up. It's a move up to your typical everyday practice without a doubt, yet kindly don't call technical support if things go amiss.

20. The Ice Bucket Challenge

Rather than dumping a can of ice water on him while you're carrying out the thing (if it's not too much trouble YouTube it, if you do), just get going in the shower. Additional credit: Melt an ice block in your mouth to chill things before giving him some frigid oral. The combo of your cool mouth and the boiling water running all over his body will be amazing.

21. The Twerk

Balancing our rundown of sex positions to attempt, we have "The Twerk." Miley Cyrus all the while advanced and destroyed twerking, yet that doesn't mean you can't at present practice it in the room. Expect the invert cowgirl position and lean forward, laying your arms on his thighs. Then basically utilize the twerking movement (curve your back and rock to and fro, popping your goods here and there) to engage in sexual relations.

Here's their guidance for removing the pressure from first-time butt-centric sex.

1. Unwind your mind...and body

The exact opposite thing you need to be before endeavoring butt-centric is tense. "If you're reluctant, anxious, or not into it, nobody will get off, and what's the purpose of that?" says Taormino. If this is your first time attempting butt-centric sex, invest some energy unwinding—clean up, request that your accomplice give you an erotic back rub, hell, you can even ponder. You can likewise concentrate on specifically loosening up your butt-centric muscles. To perceive what that feels like, fix your butt muscles—sort of like a kegel for the opposite end—and afterward discharge.

2. Convey straightforwardly

"Discussion about it first. Likewise with a wide range of sexual action, butt-centric sex is something that ought to be talked about in advance," says Needle. "Impart your apprehensions and desires with your accomplice, and ensure that you are both in the same spot about things like speed, profundity, and so forth. Trust me, this is one region in which you don't need any amazements."

All through the experience, you must focus on what you are feeling, and convey this to your accomplice. If something feels awkward or excruciating, it's dependent upon you to tell them.

3. Foam up

"Numerous ladies' dread of first-time butt-centric sex originates from a dread of what goes on back there (normally) and how that is going to play into the activity," says Needle. "To wash down yourself (actually) of such mental barriers, take a decent, hot shower first."

4. Take part in a lot of foreplay

Probably the most ideal approaches to slide into butt-centric sex is to ensure you're incredibly excited in advance. "The main misstep individuals make is surging," says Taormino. Start with foreplay, vaginal sex, whatever turns you on. (Being a couple of climaxes profound before you attempt any butt-centric infiltration helps.) "The more stirred you are, the more loosened up your sphincter muscle will be, and that is going to make for a more blazing and simpler experience," she says.

5. Utilize a ton of grease

In contrast to the vagina, the rear-end doesn't deliver its own oil. The more lube you use, the more agreeable and charming butt-centric sex can be, clarifies Needle. Remember to ensure you are utilizing a condom-safe, water or silicone-based grease (oil-based ointments aren't perfect with condoms). Try not to be reluctant to reapply oftentimes. More lube rises to better butt-centric sex consistently.

6. Expect the correct position

Three ideal positions for first-time butt-centric sex include:

You on top. It permits you to control the speed and profundity of entrance, which is critical, particularly for secondary passage beginners.

Spooning. Another extraordinary pick for secondary passage tenderfoots, this position gives you shared control of your developments and includes an additional bit of closeness, which may enable you to unwind too.

Doggy-style. This position permits your accomplice simple passage yet in addition places them in full control, which probably won't be the best for your first time.

If you feel torment anytime, have your accomplice back off, stop, or switch positions.

7. Go slowly

Regardless of how much lube you use, your indirect access isn't a water slide. First-time butt-centric sex ought to be moved toward like getting into an extremely hot bath. First you try things out during foreplay, permitting your accomplice to delicately rub around the opening with their finger, before exploring different avenues regarding really embeddings anything. Regardless of whether you're utilizing a penis, a finger, or a toy, start gradually with simply the tip before embeddings anything any more profound. The key here is to be delicate and convey. If anytime things get excessively awkward, shout out.

8. Make sure to relax

In those initial couple of seconds of infiltration, the constrain will in general reason ladies to hold their breath. This outcomes in the prompt fixing of those muscles, which will just prompt agony. Take profound, even breaths and spotlight on loosening up your whole body and discharge all strain. It might feel like you need to go to the restroom from the start, yet simply go with it.

9. Utilize a condom

Because there's no danger of getting pregnant, doesn't mean you can skirt the condom—they're the best way to forestall sexually transmitted diseases. Simply don't go from butt-centric to vaginal infiltration with a similar condom as that can spread contaminations. Dump the condom and put on another one preceding infiltrating the vagina.

10. Remember vaginal incitement

There are many mutual nerve endings between the dividers of the vagina and the butt, so animating the vagina at the same time can be incredibly pleasurable. If you feel great, embed something (maybe a finger or a vibrator) into your vagina while you are taking part in butt-centric play.

11. Try not to worry over it

If you pondering when is the perfect time to take part in first-time butt-centric sex, recall that there's no set in stone answer. For certain ladies, butt-centric sex are a no-go and for others it's a chance. Whichever way is an OK.

ADVANCED SEX POSITIONS OF KAMA SUTRA

Routine sex can slaughter a relationship, particularly if you've been with your accomplice for quite a long time. That is the reason we're here to assist you with lifting your sex game with a couple of cutting edge Kama Sutra positions:

1. The Erotic V

To get this position perfectly, you may need to invest some energy at the rec center because your legs will consume in the wake of lovemaking! Locate a table and sit on the edge. Have your person position himself before you with his legs bowed so he can infiltrate. Put your arms around his neck, and sit your privilege and left leg on his shoulders. Presently, as Fat Joe sings, recline, so he (your man, not Fat Joe — except if he puts a smile on your face) can find a workable pace.

2. The Catherine Wheel

Whoever thought of this position is a thrill seeker — and likely slammed a lady named Catherine. Start off by sitting inverse of one another. When in position, fold your legs over his middle, that is when his boa constrictor infiltrates. He then folds one leg around your hip and holds you set up. If you're not cautious, you may lose your equalization and break his penis! Hold yourself up with two hands as he directs your hips and rocks your reality like Catherine.

3. The Ape

Get bestial with The Ape — a Kama Sutra sex position that requires a tumbler. Not so much, however you do need to be extra adaptable. Here's the means by which it works: Your person lies on his back and pulls his knees to his chest. You then sit on his penis, sliding it inside gradually while propping yourself up. It's ideal for more profound entrance, however it is difficult. One bogus move and — snap!

4. The Bridge

London Bridge better not tumble down when you attempt this sex position. The breakdown may very well slaughter your hombre! That is because he should be very adaptable. Think yogi. He begins by making the state of "a scaffold" with his body. You then straddle him and sit on his Johnson. Drop the weight from of your feet so you're not smashing his masculinity. Then, werk those hips on him — and ensure he doesn't drop from the blood hurrying through his head.

5. The Seduction

I used to sit on my knees for a considerable length of time. Presently, I need to change my position at regular intervals or my legs nod off. This position isn't for me, however if you're knees are as spry as a twenty-year-olds, give it a go! To begin with, start off on your knees and lean right back. The bundles of your feet ought to be under your goods. Raise your arms over your head. Your man then lies on you, legs straight, and shimmies his way into your vagina — and the temptation starts!

6. The Dolphin

Strengthen those back muscles, you're going to require them for The Dolphin. Lie on your back and curve your back while holding yourself up by the shoulders. Your thighs and hips ought to be raised toward the roof. Keep your head and neck level. Your person then slides in the middle of your knees and lifts your hips while he's inside you. He gradually bumps you while checking your heartbeat. Joking.

7. The Plow

It's a great opportunity to get furrowed — actually. Start off on your knees before your bed. With the assistance of your person, lift yourself up onto the edge of the bed with your elbows. Fix your legs totally. Have him hold you up and step in the middle of your legs. With your hips lifted, he infiltrates. Presently, imagine yourself as a tractor and find a good pace!

Sex can in some cases get exhausting in the room doing likewise routine preacher. Fusing new sex positions and moves can bring back that pizzazz in your sexual life. Experimentation is the way to open the entryway to sexual energy and offer section to snapshots of sexual joy, erotica and climax. Your sex life may as of now be hot and zesty and chomping at the bit to go. Be that as it may, it doesn't damage to keep up the steam with experimentation of these sex positions. So here is an ace class on 10 propelled sex positions to enjoy with your accomplice for electrifying sex.

This is an interpretation of the mainstream sex position – the Missionary. It is a propelled adaptation of the preacher. To play out this sex position the lady needs to lay on her back like in the Missionary and spread her legs separated while the man positions himself over her. Rather than putting her spread legs on the bed, the lady pulls them closer to her chest and spots them on the man's shoulders with the goal that her calves or lower legs are laying on his shoulders on either side of his neck. Thus the name – The Anvil. To give him inconceivable delight the lady can give him an oral in the Anvil position as her mouth is nearer to his penis. In spite of the fact that the man appears in charge right now, really the lady can control how profound he enters by pushing him off with her legs till she discover a spot which gives her sexual joy. The two accomplices should be adaptable and fit to complete this situation as it includes utilizing the quality of calf and thigh muscles for holding in position. If the man's penis is too long it tends to be excruciating during infiltration right now.

2. The Catherine Wheel or Pinwheel

This is a Kamasutra progressed and entangled sex position. The man and lady sit confronting one another. The man enters the lady right now the lady folds her legs over his middle while entrance. The lady underpins herself with her hands on the bed or floor while reclining. The man presently traverses one leg over her to secure her while supporting himself on one elbow. So as to push, the lady can push with her arms, and the man can manage the development with his hands on her abdomen or knees. This sex position permits entrance profound into the vagina giving most extreme sexual joy to the lady. Right now man has one hand allowed to animate the clitoris, contact the bosoms or other foreplay. The two accomplices have the joy of looking at one another without flinching during the lovemaking demonstration. This position includes moderate and sexy sex prompting orgasmic delight gradually and consistently. Nobody accomplice controls right now.

3. V is for Vixen or the Erotic V

The suggestive V is a sex position that gets its name from the situation of the lady during intercourse. The lady sits on the edge of a table at a level with the end goal that the man is in a position agreeable enough to enter her. She presently spreads her legs and reclines. His legs ought to be marginally twisted and divided somewhat separated. When the man enters, she puts her major advantages over his shoulders. She can bolster herself by either folding her arms over his neck for help or reclining with her arms on the table. This position considers extremely profound infiltration. The position likewise permits the man to pet the lady's bosoms and kiss her which without a doubt expands the delight remainder. This sensual sex position can be utilized homosexual and lesbian couples also. Homosexual men can utilize this situation as a variety of butt-centric sex, while lesbian couples can utilize a lash on dildo to accomplish entrance.

4. The 69

Ladies like accepting oral sex as much as men. The man gives delight while alluring her to satisfy him as well. 69 is a situation wherein the two accomplices are commonly transformed and perform oral sex on one another simultaneously. It tends to be performed both with man on top or the lady on top. Performing it in a sideways position is simpler. 69 requires skilful coordination and situating between the couples to make it sexually pleasurable. 69 is an incredible sex position to knock up the sexual meter when sex begins getting exhausting and tedious. Since the two accomplices perform oral sex on one another at same time it is an efficient position. In any case, if one accomplices climaxes before the other it can hose the sexual rush totally. Men for the most part discharge quicker and consequently the man ought to enjoy foreplay and work on the lady some time before the lady begins on him.

5. Joystick Joyride

This is like a lady on top position. The man lies on his back with his arms loose over his head. The lady rides him to such an extent that her feet are on either sides of his shoulder. The lady causes the man to enter her with his penis and afterward begins swiveling her hips in to and fro, here and there and turning developments simply like a gaming joystick. She step by step expands the rhythm and the extent of the developments. While she is swiveling, her boobs move every which way including visual joy for the man. This sex position has the lady completely in charge of the speed, heading and power, leaving the man allowed to unwind and appreciate. The man's hands are allowed to stroke the lady's bosoms and invigorate her clitoris. This position is extraordinary for G spot incitement.

6. The Bridge

The Bridge is a propelled sex position which requires a solid and adaptable male accomplice practically like a yogi. The man brings himself up in the extension position angling his back with his feet and turns in an all-encompassing position. The lady straddles across him and sits on his dick ensuring she doesn't rest the whole weight of her body on him by dropping the weight from her feet. An activity ball can be utilized to help a looser type of the Bridge. Spot the activity ball under the male accomplice has returned to help him if his quality gives out. Upon entrance the lady pushes every which way expanding sexual joy. Right now, the man gets a corkscrew sensation while the lady finds a good pace control.

7. The Plow

Athletic, adaptable and solid couples can enjoy this propelled sex position. The lady lies on the bed looking down with the end goal that are hips are on the edge and her legs are off the bed. While she bolsters herself on her elbows the man enters from between her legs which are loosened up behind her, lifts up her hips and thighs and enters from behind. This difficult sex position takes into consideration better entrance and more noteworthy G-spot incitement. Additionally, it helps increment the odds of pregnancy.

8. The Seduction

This position needs the administrations of an adaptable female accomplice who stoops with her back on the bed and her feet tucked under her goods and hands over her head. The man enters the lady from the top with his legs together and bolsters his weight on his lower arms which are laid on the bed on either side of the lady's middle. A few females discover leaving one leg tucked under her base and the other loosened up straight progressively agreeable. This position can be very pleasurable for the lady however she should be profoundly adaptable. This position can cause a lady to feel just as she is alluring her accomplice by showing herself so provocatively, which can be very exciting without anyone else. Furthermore, this position tilts a woman's pelvis upward marginally, which can help encourage clitoral incitement during intercourse, prompting simpler and increasingly extraordinary female climaxes.

9. The Ape

The lady can get carnal with her man with the Ape sex position. The man lies on his back with knees pulled near chest. The lady sits in reverse on the rear of his thighs and slides his penis into her vagina while propping herself facing his feet. Try to incline toward his legs and hold his wrists or then prop herself up on the bed or floor to make the position agreeable and afterward push. This sex position holds useful for butt-centric sex as well. Right now penis enters profound, contacting the vaginal divider giving the lady a mind boggling sexual sensation.

10. The Waterfall

The lady rests on her back with hips on the edge of the bed and her head and shoulders on the floor while the man moves to the edge of the bed and enters her from the top. The head being lower than the body there is a surge of blood through the head giving the lady an astounding inclination. The point of the vaginal divider is currently flawlessly situated for his penis to rub her G spot while he gets a super-tight treat. The positions of the couple can be exchanged too with the male on the floor and the lady in the top position.

11. The Clasp

In the Clasp, the couple stand confronting each other with the lady's back upheld by a divider. While she spreads her legs he curves and enters from the front. While hunching down he snatches the lady with the end goal that her legs are twisted around his midriff. He then stands up pushing the lady towards the divider while infiltrating and pushing her simultaneously. This position is perfect for sex whenever anyplace. Nonetheless, it requires a specific level of solidarity from the man and lady both.

Try not to take the propelled sex ace class too truly. Have some good times testing the different sex positions to get close and bond with your accomplice. Evaluating these sex positions isn't simple and you may not look sexy, hot or fabulous either. Be that as it may, what the hell! Entertain yourselves and have a shaking throbbing night!

BEST SEX POSITION DURING PREGNANCY

Because let's be honest — it's not generally that agreeable

Along these lines, you probably won't have the option to have intercourse in the teacher position for a while, yet that is OK. There's a lot of other sexual positions you can pull off for that post-climax sparkle.

All things considered, sex is tied in with appreciating the body, closeness, and closeness. Furthermore, if you're stressed penetrative sex may hurt the child (it won't), there are as yet different ways around that!

"Sex is significantly more than entrance," affirms Holly Richmond, a clinical sex advisor and authorized marriage and family specialist. Closeness comes in a lot of structures, including kissing, bosom delight, oral sex, dream, and even butt-centric sex.

"Oral and manual [acts finished with your hands] sex are awesome segments to a couple's sex life. Find out about oral sex strategies. Play with some new toys. If anything doesn't feel right, ask your PCP."

Positions to maintain a strategic distance from

Preacher position (man on top, lady on base) can pack blood stream to mother and child, especially after the twentieth week.

A few ladies find inclined positions, or lying level on the stomach, awkward.

As verified by each specialist and pregnancy book you'll at any point read, don't explode air there.

Consider pregnancy an opportunity to analyze, particularly in the previous months, to make sense of the perfect situation among you and your accomplice. What's more, basically anything goes as long as it's agreeable.

In any case, you may have inquiries regarding how to modify for greatest stomach comfort when connecting with your accomplice. We'll walk you through it — with visuals!

1. Sex from behind

This position is frequently refered to by sex instructors as a well-known choice for a wide range of accomplices. Up down on the ground, this position keeps pressure off the gut, permitting the pregnant accomplice to remain increasingly agreeable.

"Utilizing cushions, covers, or towels to include comfort is an extraordinary thought," says Shanna Katz Kattari, a sexologist and educator at the University of Michigan School of Social Work.

Controlling the profundity of entrance is likewise significant, Richmond calls attention to. "Now and then in that position with the arch of the back, [the pregnant partner] can feel the penis hitting the cervix," which might be awkward.

Trimester: First and start of second. Before the second's over trimester, there's about an additional two pounds around your midsection. You might need to abstain from adjusting down on the ground during your most recent two months.

2. You on top

Move on board! This position is bolstered by science, as well — at any rate one Taiwanese examination discovered expanded sexual fulfillment for pregnant ladies who control infiltration by being on the accomplice.

Modify for comfort by augmenting your position or reclining to keep paunch weight from tilting you forward.

Trimester: First and second trimester. This position assists with hitting the correct spots in the vagina. In any case, during the third trimester, you might need to stay away from profound infiltration, particularly if you're delicate down there and need to abstain from aggravating the cervix or unplanned dying.

3. Spooning sex

"Spooning is great," Richmond says. It's an ameliorating position where the accomplice holds and as a rule infiltrates the pregnant accomplice from behind while resting, both confronting endlessly from one another.

In any case, regardless of whether you're infiltrating or not, generally contact the clitoris as that is the place the joy community may be. In later trimesters, it might be consoling to hold the paunch.

Trimester: Always great, however best during second and third as this position can help put less focus on the paunch.

4. Turn around cowgirl

Turn around cowgirl includes you, or the pregnant accomplice, straddling the other and is a decent alternative in the first and second trimesters, Richmond says. Make certain to keep up the clitoral incitement right now.

Be that as it may, it very well may be testing later on when your midsection turns into a test. If this position is one of your top picks, you might have the option to modify the weight by reclining and situating your arms behind you for help.

Trimester: Great whenever, however during the second and third trimesters, you'll love this situation as it can shield your stomach from being packed — or contacted, if you're delicate there.

5. Standing

If under 20 weeks, a standing position works if your accomplice is holding you around the midsection.

"Following 20 weeks, the stomach enlargement could cause more offset issues and difficulty with position," she says, which represents a danger of falling. The pregnant accomplice may put palms against a divider, and lean in for solidness. In any case, look for strong ground.

"I don't prescribe remaining on anything, again for security and strength purposes," she says. "No yoga obstructs, no seats, no stepping stools."

Trimester: Experiment with this during the first and second trimesters, however as your midsection develops, you may think that its progressively difficult to hold this position. If it's pleasurable for your accomplice, you could figure out how to fuse it close to the finish of intercourse.

6. Drifting pregnant position

"A pregnant individual may appreciate sex in the bath, where they can drift while giving or getting delight," Katz Kattari says. Lightness enables a tummy to resist gravity — a pleasant choice when you're 8 months along.

Contingent upon the size of your tub, you will most likely be unable to drift totally, so your accomplice can support the experience. Have them lie under you for help and let their hands invigorate your touchy zones for joy. If utilizing toys, make certain to utilize water-safe lube.

Trimester: This works for all trimesters. Be that as it may, during the third trimester, when you're increasingly delicate and charisma is low, this position is a soothing one where climaxes don't need to be the end game. This can essentially simply be tied in with thinking about one another in an exotic manner.

7. Situated pregnancy sex

Couples of numerous kinds can appreciate situated intercourse, where the pregnant individual sits on a seat or on the edge of the bed, situating themselves over their accomplice. You can likewise prop yourself up with cushions, or lie on your back prior in pregnancy, or if agreeable.

"Their accomplice would then be able to have simple access for fingers, toys, and mouths," Katz Kattari says. "Either by bowing before pregnant individual, or finding a comfortable place to sit beside them and getting down to business."

8. Pregnant oral sex

Indeed, giving or getting oral sex is fine, says Aleece Fosnight, MSPAC, PA-C, CSC, CSE. It doesn't make a difference if you swallow if you're giving oral sex to a collaborate with a penis — it won't influence the infant. What's more, if you're getting oral sex, it won't influence the creating infant, particularly in the last trimester.

Additionally, it's a wonderful option in contrast to penetrative sex if you're only not available. In any case, if giving oral sex to a cooperate with a penis, know that during the main trimester, you may have an increased stifler reflex because of morning ailment.

Trimester: Good for all trimesters, in any event, when you're not pregnant. While clitoral incitement is one of the more solid ways to climax, not all sex needs to end in a climax. Sex is about physical closeness, regardless of whether there's entrance or not, or climaxes or not.

9. Butt-centric sex

Truly, butt-centric sex is sheltered during pregnancy and can be performed with your accomplice at your back or while spooning. Doggy style, or entering from behind, would be the best for butt-centric sex during pregnancy. You can likewise do this while spooning as well.

It's ideal if you attempt this position at an early stage, before pregnancy, to perceive how agreeable you are with butt-centric sex.

Butt-centric sex proposals

Go slow and get ready with foreplay for in any event 10 to 15 minutes.

Use lube, particularly during pregnancy.

Wear a condom for additional assurance against microorganisms and STIs.

Trimester: This position works for all trimesters. Notwithstanding, you'll need to be incredibly cautious. Try not to move fingers, toys, tongue, or penis from butt to vagina. Doing so can spread microbes to the vagina, which could muddle pregnancy.

10. Next to each other sex

It's like spooning, with the exception of you're confronting one another.

"For any pregnant individual, positions on their side will feel much improved, and they can prop up their paunches with additional pads or a moved up towel," Katz Kattari says. "These side positions can be utilized for penetrative sex with hands and toys, just as for both giving and getting oral sex."

Which means you can pivot and attempt 69 if that is something you like.

Trimester: Good for all, best for third as it takes into account you or your pregnant accomplice to lay on your sides without squeezing the stomach — or on one another!

Open the joybox

If you're not feeling excessively hot or up for foreplay, there's additionally a mystical wand you can wave — the one with batteries.

"Top toys consistently incorporate the Magic Wand and the Wevibe," says Rosara Torrisi, a sex specialist and originator of the Long Island Institute of Sex Therapy.

"All toys, inasmuch as the materials are body sheltered and high caliber and cleaned suitably, are protected during pregnancy except if in any case coordinated by a believed clinical expert who knows you and your pregnancy."

So yes — vibrators, dildos, insertables, balls, G-spot triggers, tie ons and whatever else you have in your joybox is fine, as long as you keep hardware very extra astonishing clean.

If you're purchasing new props, expect to get one produced using higher-grade materials, for example, glass, silicone, or body-safe latex.

Because of clitoral affectability, you may wish to play with power and speed. A few ladies locate the Magic Wand and other powerful vibrators excessively extraordinary, Richmond says.

CONCLUSION

So which of the Kama Sutra Positions can fulfill your ladies colossally and help her to accomplish various climaxes? Ladies presently are progressively worried about having sexual fulfillment, and how they are treated when sex.

In the Kama Sutra manual, there are a variety of systems, abilities, and manners that are fundamentals for you to know if you need to fulfill her in bed. Sex ought not simply end with climax and discharge as this will just leave ladies to feel disappointed and void.

All the different Kama Sutra Positions have the potential outcomes to fulfill your darling incredibly, however everything relies upon whether you are eager to investigate new positions and strategies. Let me simply share with you extraordinary compared to other Kama Sutra positions that can cause her to go wild:

The Widely Opened Position. This position begins with the lady resting with her back curved, head tossed back and body raised to meet her accomplice spreading her legs wide giving a point of passage to guarantee profound infiltration.

This position gives more fulfillment to the lady then the man as the private parts comes into contact. This is because this position gives her clitoris full presentation to the grating of the intercourse. In any case, he may basically miss the sentiment of the tight control as she shuts her legs against his penis.

The man can bolster himself by propping his himself up with his arms. The lady should keep her body curved to meet her darling and investigate his eyes to build the degree of closeness.

You can give your ladies sexual fulfillment today. Sex is a piece of your life, and you should make each meeting of it be a satisfying and pleasant one.

Printed in Great Britain
by Amazon